Breaking Barriers

ADVANCES IN COMMUNITY PSYCHOLOGY SERIES

The Book Series of the Society for Community Research and Action

Series Editor
Robin Lin Miller

Advisory Board
Nicole Allen
Valerie Anderson
Anne Bogat
Scotney D. Evans
Shabnam Javdani
Bret Kloos
Kien Lee
Eric Mankowski
Kenneth I. Maton
José H. Ornelas
Isaac Prilleltensky
Manuel Riemer
Bernadette Sanchez
Marybeth Shinn
Nathan Todd
Blanca Ortiz Torres
Judah J. Viola
Roderick Watts
Bianca D. M. Wilson

Books in the Series
Principles of Social Change
Leonard A. Jason

Community Psychology and Community Mental Health: Towards Transformative Change
Edited by Geoffrey Nelson, Bret Kloos, and José H. Ornelas

Influencing Social Policy: Applied Psychology Serving the Public Interest
Kenneth I. Maton

Housing, Citizenship, and Communities for People with Serious Mental Illness: Theory, Research, Practice, and Policy Perspectives
Edited by John Sylvestre, Geoffrey Nelson, and Tim Aubry

Diverse Careers in Community Psychology
Edited by Judah J. Viola and Olya Glantsman

Community Power and Empowerment
Brian D. Christens

Breaking Barriers: Sexual and Gender Minority-Led Advocacy to End AIDS in Africa and the Caribbean
Robin Lin Miller and George Ayala

Forthcoming Books in the Series
Rethinking American Indian Mental Health: Perspectives from Community Psychology
Joseph P. Gone

Breaking Barriers

*Sexual and Gender Minority-Led Advocacy to
End AIDS in Africa and the Caribbean*

Robin Lin Miller and George Ayala

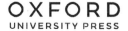

OXFORD
UNIVERSITY PRESS

OXFORD
UNIVERSITY PRESS

Oxford University Press is a department of the University of Oxford. It furthers
the University's objective of excellence in research, scholarship, and education
by publishing worldwide. Oxford is a registered trade mark of Oxford University
Press in the UK and certain other countries.

Published in the United States of America by Oxford University Press
198 Madison Avenue, New York, NY 10016, United States of America.

© Oxford University Press 2024

CIP data is on file at the Library of Congress

ISBN 978–0–19–764768–4

DOI: 10.1093/oso/9780197647684.001.0001

Printed by Marquis Book Printing, Canada

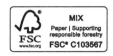

Contents

Tables and Figure

Tables

Figure

Series Foreword

The Society for Community Research and Action (SCRA), Division 27 of the American Psychological Association, is an international and interdisciplinary organization that supports the development of theory, research, and social action to promote empowerment, health, and well-being. Members give special attention to multiple levels of analysis, including the individual, group, organizational, community, cultural, and societal levels. Members focus on an array of pressing social issues within national and global contexts, such as violence, poverty, and racism, and have developed, using a continuum of frameworks from prevention to intervention to structural change, effective approaches to address seemingly intractable issues in partnership with local communities. These approaches to change involve diverse strategies, including, for example, advocacy, citizen participation, collaboration, community organizing, economic development, preventive education, self-help/mutual help, sociopolitical development, social movements, and policy change. Each typically shares the goal of challenging and altering underlying power structures in the pursuit of social justice and community and individual well-being.

This book series, Advances in Community Psychology, is sponsored by the SCRA and aims to aid in the dissemination of theory, research, and social action as developed by SCRA members, as well as nonmembers working in allied disciplines. The overarching mission of the series is to create a publication venue that (a) highlights the contributions of the field of community psychology and, more generally, community action, research, and practice; (b) integrates current knowledge regarding pressing topics and priorities for the field; and (c) offers the foundation for future directions.

After several years serving in the role of series editor, it became apparent to me (Robin) that writing a book on my own work might contribute to the mission of the series. In early 2021, in partnership with George Ayala, I developed a proposal and, in recognition of the inappropriateness of serving as the series editor of my own work, asked SCRA's Publication Chair and Book Series Editorial Board Member, Judah J. Viola, to serve as its action editor. Judah graciously agreed and oversaw the shepherding of the proposal and resulting book through to the process of its completion. This volume reflects his efforts as action editor and mine as author, while also series editor, hence we write this foreword together.

This volume in the series, *Breaking Barriers: Sexual and Gender Minority-Led Advocacy to End AIDS in Africa and the Caribbean*, provides an in-depth examination of an award-winning transnational advocacy partnership among sexual and gender minority community-led activist organizations in eight countries titled Project ACT. Project ACT aimed to remove barriers to HIV care for gay and bisexual men and transgender women in Africa and the Caribbean using advocacy strategies and tactics. Project ACT received a 2022 Exemplary Project W. K. Kellogg Foundation Community Engagement Scholarship Award from the Association of Public and Land Grant Universities and Engagement Scholarship Consortium in recognition of the transnational partnerships' contributions to improving the lives of sexual and gender minority people in multiple countries.

In *Breaking Barriers*, Robin Lin Miller and George Ayala begin by situating Project ACT within the context of the colonial and postcolonial influences that contribute to social, political, and legal exclusion that prevents sexual and gender minority people and the community-led organizations that represent their interests from full participation in civil society. They outline for the reader how this exclusion obstructs efforts to promote the sexual health and human rights of sexual and gender minority people and impedes progress in ending the HIV epidemic. They further consider how the dynamics of development funding and international partnerships impact on the ability of sexual and gender minority communities in Africa and the Caribbean to address local needs and pursue local advocacy priorities that are vital to ending AIDS.

Miller and Ayala are powerful storytellers. They invite readers to experience the day-to-day rhythms and trials of the community-led organizations as they advocate on behalf of their constituents. By showing in-depth the realities faced by these organizations and the nature of their advocacy to ensure sexual and gender minority people can access HIV care, readers develop a newfound appreciation for the role these organizations can play in advancing social change and just how hard their work can be. Through exploring the experiences of the Project ACT partners, Miller and Ayala offer readers policy and practice recommendations for removing structural barriers to HIV care for sexual and gender minority communities that are as compelling as they are practical.

Miller and Ayala deftly address the role of evaluation and engaged forms of scholarship in human rights advocacy efforts and outline the features that distinguish advocacy evaluation as a unique area of practice. They also grapple with the dilemmas faced by small community-led organizations when they are expected to demonstrate accountability to funders and the power dynamics inherent in funders' relationships to small community-led organizations. Miller and Ayala elaborate on the conceptual and methodological challenges of evaluating projects like Project ACT, giving readers an appreciation for the complexities and dilemmas of evaluating human rights advocacy initiatives in ways that are sensible, realize human rights principles, and honor local values. Their report of the project's implementation and its achievements, and of their evaluation approach, illustrate the balancing of scientific rigor and respectful engagement of the activists with whom they worked. Through their account of how they evaluated Project ACT and how that evaluation supported activists' ongoing learning, they contribute to an emergent body of literature on best practices for advocacy evaluation, as well as for community engagement and action research generally.

Throughout their retelling, Miller and Ayala locate themselves in every step of the work, illustrating the importance of positionality in research and action and revealing evaluators and action researchers as human beings. Miller served as the project's evaluator and Ayala as the Executive Director of the community-led organization that led Project ACT. By showing themselves in the book and speaking from the perspective of their roles on the project, they offer readers a fresh and nuanced account of the dynamics of community–academic partnerships. *Breaking Barriers* elegantly presents the principles of advocacy practice and effective partnerships that contributed to Project ACT's successes and challenges. We invite readers to utilize *Breaking Barriers* and apply its lessons in their own advocacy and evaluation practice. Activists, community psychologists, evaluators, HIV care providers, and funders of community-led HIV responses should consider *Breaking Barriers* compulsory reading.

Judah J. Viola, SCRA Publication Chair and Editorial Board Member

Robin Lin Miller, Series Editor

Acknowledgments

We owe an immeasurable debt to the activists and allies who were willing to take on the advocacy work that we describe in this book and to those who so graciously welcomed Robin and MPact staff members into their organizations each time they appeared on their doorstep. We learned and accomplished more than we could have ever imagined from closely observing and supporting their efforts to improve the lives of their community members. We are humbled by their wisdom, courage, and candor.

Writing our first book presented us with a steep learning curve about the world of book publishing. We owe special thanks to John Sibley Williams, who gently guided us through the contracting process, and coached us on how to develop a thoughtful marketing strategy. We are forever grateful to Robin's writing coach, Katey Schultz, for sharing her incredibly smart approaches to deep revision and her sage advice on how to obtain useful feedback during the writing process. At every stage of our writing process, we have benefited from thoughtful reviews. We received anonymous reviews of our initial book proposal from four colleagues and of the penultimate draft of the manuscript from two additional colleagues. We appreciate these reviewers' excitement about our work and the useful suggestions that they made. Judah Viola also provided us with helpful guidance as we set out to compose our first draft. We are indebted to each of these colleagues for the many ways in which they helped us make this book a better one. Kim Greenwell and James McMillen provided us with a masterful developmental edit of the manuscript as it neared its final stages. We cannot say enough about the ways in which they helped us to express our ideas with greater clarity and precision.

We heeded the counsel of several veteran writers, including Katey Schultz, who urged us to assemble a panel of critical friends to read along as we produced our first draft of this book and share their impressions. Our critical friends were incredibly generous to do this for us. The discussions we held with these friends provided us with a roadmap to revision and helped us identify more clearly why we wrote and for whom. We believe our book is immeasurably improved thanks to their cogent insights and honest appraisals: Anne Coghlan, Laurel Sprague, and Marc Zimmerman.

It probably would not have occurred to either of us to write this book in the way that we did, had not Robin's dear friend, and a mentor to so many of us in community psychology, Edison J. Trickett, repeatedly called for stories that take researchers under the hood of research projects like ours; to show ourselves doing the work and reflecting on our action. Ed had agreed to be among our critical friend readers, but he passed away unexpectedly in May 2022 while we were in the process of our initial drafting. We honor him for his inspiration to embark on this task. We hope that we have satisfactorily balanced his wish for more first-person accounts of community psychologists in action against our desire to place the community-led activists with whom we were privileged to collaborate on Project ACT in the forefront.

Other critical friends joined in as we went along, even hosting us at their homes when revising the book required that we isolate ourselves in their guest rooms. We are forever grateful to Susan Tucker, who welcomed us to invade her home for a 4-day writing retreat. Her dining table is where much of our revision work happened. And to Pato Hebert, who generously engaged in critical discussions with George about the book's organization, title, significance, and the dynamics of co-authoring, even as they were working together on their own book. The inspiration and support provided by Susan and Pato were invaluable.

The evaluation of Project ACT was made possible by many people at Michigan State University, who dedicated their time and expertise to ensure it was a successful process. These included people who assisted in translating and back-translating materials, developing a data safety plan, and processing mountains of travel receipts. We are especially grateful to Tatiana Bustos, Rosaura Dominguez, David Figueroamartin, Jean Kayitsinga, and Jack Wehyrich for their document translation assistance; to Chip Shank for his co-investigation of global information technology security issues and help in data safety plan development; to Joe Cesario for pointing us down productive pathways in the social psychology literature that helped us better understand our data; and, to Jan Reaume and Nick Drew for their help with navigating oodles of regulations and procedures governing everything from budgets to travel, and for their seemingly endless patience. Every time Robin returned from a data gathering trip, she faced the daunting task of transcribing hours of audio recordings into text. An army of undergraduate and graduate student volunteers from Michigan State University assisted in this process: Sarah Alabdali, Rachael Bailey, Maeve Denshaw, Gabrielle Grace, Brynn Muehlenberg, Alex Pawalaczyk, Zoe Pride, Sarah Raider, Zach Sebree, Rachel Weber, Cameron Wilson, and Fangzhou Xu. It was not easy under ideal circumstances, and proved a very tedious, lonely task during COVID-19 lockdowns. We could not fully capture the voices and language of those who shared their experiences and perspectives with Robin without these students' help. Training, supervising, and cheering on all these talented students was an amazing graduate student, Jaleah Rutledge. Jaleah also conducted virtual interviews and assisted Robin in the analysis of our outcome data. Her orientation to detail and her insightfulness each proved indispensable. The interviews conducted in the Francophone countries that Robin visited were assisted by three translators, two of whom are known in this book as Chantal and Laurent, and a third, who we will call here Prince. Each merits an honorary certificate in evaluation (seriously!) and earned Robin's undying gratitude and admiration.

Nothing about this project would have occurred without the unwavering commitment to MPact's mission shown by Lily May Catanes, Johnasies McGraw, Sherrie Hicks, and Zamora. Their handling of logistics, finance, and so much more for Project ACT made retreats in Cambodia and Rwanda appear seamless. Angel Fabian also helped move the project forward, with their brilliant questions and terrific ideas. But the heart and soul of the project were the six brilliant activists who worked shoulder to shoulder with love, humor, and unflagging dedication: Omar Baños, Stephen Leonelli, Nadia Rafif, Mohan Sundararaj, Greg Tartaglione, and Johnny Tohme. Robin is humbled to be a member of the extended Project ACT family. And George couldn't be prouder.

Project ACT would also not have occurred were it not for the Elton John AIDS Foundation's willingness to establish a funding mechanism, in partnership with the Office of the United States' Global AIDS Coordinator, to support this type of LGBT activism. Although we are candid in this book about our interactions with the Foundation, we are eternally grateful for their willingness to lend financial support to the work we describe. Their support is incredibly brave and all too rare. It is also essential to realizing human rights for LGBT people. We will not bring an end to AIDS in the parts of the world where it is difficult to create the enabling environments on which ending the epidemic depends, without more funding institutions following the Foundation's leadership.

MPact pushed its way into the world and, in turn, delivered Project ACT and dozens of initiatives like it. MPact was shouldered by scores of visionaries who understood the vital role it played in ensuring LGBT people were heard by and visible to those who occupied positions of power. These brilliant lights in the universe must be named with deference and appreciation. They include Cornelius Baker, Don Baxter, Aditya Bondyopadhyay, Richard Burzynski, Gus Cairns, Robert Carr, Simón Cazal, Ton Coenen, Carlos García de León, Juan Jacobo Hernández, Paul Jansen, Rapeepun Ohm Jommaroeng, JoAnne Keatley, Shivananda Khan, Tudor Kovacs, Zhen Li, Samuel Matzikure, John Maxwell, Othman Mellouk, Ken Morrison, Joel Nana, Steave Nemande, Midnight Poonkasetwattana, Andy Quan, Leonardo Sánchez, Paul Semugoma, Ruth Morgan Thomas, Craig Thompson, and the original MPact secretariat. To the many people we forgot to mention, we hold you in our hearts and in the spirit of this book.

We owe a special debt to Robin's partner, Miles McNall. Miles deserves a prize for having read draft after draft after draft of every chapter. His contributions appear on every single page, whether those pages made it into the book or fell to the cutting room floor at his urging. Miles served as a sounding board for Robin's thinking about how to design and manage the evaluation throughout. He put up with the many long absences that conducting the evaluation required, complaining only a little about walking the dog alone rather than together, as is the evening ritual. Robin's son, Evan, too, tolerated these absences and disruptions to his life, routinely cheering the project and its team on. Travelling to IAS with the team for the 2018 conference, he offered trenchant observations of IAS and its power dynamics, insights that struck us deeply. George's life partner, Đỗ Đăng Trị, also deserves our special appreciation. Trị stood steadfast, patiently supporting George as he logged countless hours away from home. Trị stood ready to supply that long, loving embrace that a travel-weary and work-beaten George needed. Trị was (and still is) a rock-steady companion and thought partner. A silent but powerful and insightful influence, Trị was as much a part of

MPact's development as George was. Thank you, Miles, Evan, and Trị, for loving, supporting, and holding home for us.

Writing a book is an intimate act. We spent hundreds of hours together taking chapters apart, scrutinizing each word, and unpacking every idea. We explored, discussed, and deliberated over several years. And we listened. We listened to community activists as they generously offered testimony. We gently listened to each other. We supported each other through uncertainty, chronic disease, and personal loss. Through it all, the book served as an anchor. Through the process of its creation, we grew to understand one another and ourselves more deeply as writers, as researchers, as community psychologists, as human rights advocates, and as people. There are no words that could express the respect and appreciation we feel for one another, a debt we owe in no small part to the process of creating this book together.

Abbreviations

ART	Antiretroviral therapy
COP	Country Operational Plan
CSO	Community-service organization
EJAF	Elton John AIDS Foundation
GALZ	Gays and Lesbians of Zimbabwe
The Global Fund	The Global Fund to Fight AIDS, Tuberculosis, and Malaria
GMHC	Gay Men's Health Crisis
HAART	Highly active antiretroviral therapy
IAS	International AIDS Society
ICASA	International Conference on AIDS and STIs in Africa
IRB	Institutional Review Board
LGBT	Lesbian, gay, bisexual, and transgender
LGBTQIA	Lesbian, gay, bisexual, transgender, queer, intersex, asexual
M&E	Monitoring and evaluation
MPACT	MPact Global Action for Gay Men's Health and Rights
MSM	Men who have sex with men
MSMGF	The Global Forum on MSM and HIV
MSMIT	Implementing Comprehensive HIV and STI Program with Men who have Sex with Men: Practical Guidance for Collaborative Interventions
NGO	Nongovernment organization
OGAC	Office of the Global AIDS Coordinator
PEPFAR	United States President's Emergency Plan for AIDS Relief
Project ACT	Advocacy and other community tactics
PSI	Population Services International
RSAT	Rainbow Sky Association for Thailand
SRC	Sexual Rights Centre
UKAID	United Kingdom Agency for International Development
UNAIDS	The Joint United Nations Program on HIV/AIDS
USAID	United States Agency for International Development
U = U	Undetectable equals untransmittable
WHO	World Health Organization

Project ACT Timeline

July 2004	Don Baxter and others begin organizing a global network of gay and bisexual men HIV activists.
July 2006	The Global Forum on MSM and HIV (now known as MPact Global Action for Gay Men's Health and Rights) is founded.
November 2010	Preliminary results from the IPrex trial are published in the *New England Journal of Medicine*. Results support the efficacy of pre-exposure prophylaxis.
July 2012	The International AIDS Conference is held in the United States for the first time in more than 20 years. Secretary of State Hillary Rodham Clinton is among the plenary speakers.
November 2014	168 nations agree to a fast-track strategy to end AIDS by 2030. As part of that agreement, midterm targets are established to ensure 90% of people living with HIV know their HIV status, 90% are treated, and 90% achieve viral suppression.
June 2016	The Elton John AIDS Foundation announces the establishment of the LGBT Fund in partnership with the United States Office of the Global AIDS Coordinator.
July 2016	The inaugural recipients of LGBT Fund awards are announced at the International AIDS Conference in Durban, South Africa. MPact receives a small grant to remove barriers to HIV care in Africa and the Caribbean.
August 2016–November 2017	MPact begins identifying partners and conceptualizing Project ACT.
April 2018	MPact receives the LGBT Fund award promised to it in 2016. MPact hosts a preliminary overview webinar for partners identified to date.
May 2018	Robin joins the Project ACT team. The final Project ACT partners are identified.
June 2018	MPact hosts Project ACT kickoff meeting in Siem Riep, Cambodia.
July 2018	MPact convenes the "Out with It" pre-conference at International AIDS Conference in Amsterdam. Plenary speakers at the main conference acknowledge the 90-90-90 targets will not be met.
August 2018	Advocacy begins in some Project ACT countries.
December 2018	Evaluation data collection of Project ACT officially begins in Jamaica. Rainbow House in Jamaica burns down. The Polyplas Factor in the Dominican Republic explodes.

January 2019	Zimbabwe is rocked by riots and hyperinflation. MPact holds its annual strategic planning retreat.
January–March 2019	Initial evaluation visits to Zimbabwe, Cameroon, Côte d'Ivoire.
April 2019	MPact staff review first round of evaluation data in an all-staff reflective session.
June 2019	LGBT Fund withholds funds.
July–August 2019	Second data collection visits to Zimbabwe, Cameroon, Côte d'Ivoire.
September 2019	Second data collection visit to Jamaica.
December 2019	Project ACT partners gather in Rwanda for a final reflection and lessons learned workshop.
February–March 2020	Final data collection visits to Cameroon and Côte d'Ivoire.
March 2020	Final data collection visits to Jamaica and Zimbabwe cancelled due to COVID-19 pandemic. Supplementary data collection to Ghana also cancelled.
August 2020	Project ACT team holds last reflection meeting.
October 2020	George steps down from the helm of MPact.

Introduction

Avenir Jeune de L'Ouest

On the evening of April 20, 2018, not long after sunset, three employees of Avenir Jeune de L'Ouest—its executive director, its warden, and a health care worker—were arrested at their headquarters by two plainclothes police officers.[1] The officers had no warrant and, by some reports, provided no identification to verify that they were policemen. Two further staff members were arrested at their homes the following morning. In the months preceding the arrests, harassment directed at the Avenir Jeune de L'Ouest staff by anonymous sources, including death threats, had become as common as the thunderstorms that prowl Cameroon's evening skies. Eight months of reporting the ongoing harassment to police garnered no response. Perhaps, the staff reasoned, disregard for their safety was a predictable hazard of serving their members. Or maybe they suspected the police were the more formidable antagonist so declined to press the issue of their neglected complaints.

The police detained the five men at Dschang's Central Police Station for 4 days before granting them access to legal representation. During one of several interrogations while they were held in custody, an officer reportedly disclosed that Avenir Jeune de L'Ouest and its workers had been under surveillance for some time. Eventually, the men learned they were apprehended on suspicion of homosexuality, which under Cameroon's penal code (Article 347-1) carries a potential prison term of up to 5 years and a fine of up to US$360.

During their imprisonment, the five men were confined to a single cell without a bed or sanitary facilities. They slept on the floor and shared one bucket between them. They lacked access to clean water. Although it is only legal to detain citizens for 48 hours uncharged, the men waited a week in jail—until their lawyer, aided by international supporters, secured their release on bail. A small victory. But the judge who granted their release ordered the men to return to the police station for rectal examinations within the week—a humiliating procedure, and medically useless for its claimed purpose of establishing homosexuality. Thanks to their lawyer's continued intervention, the judge ultimately rescinded this order.

Avenir Jeune de L'Ouest received such intense police scrutiny because it serves lesbian, gay, bisexual, and transgender (LGBT) people[2] living with HIV, and advocates for their rights, a tiny yet welcome respite in a landscape of unwelcoming mainstream alternatives. Avenir Jeune de l'Ouest is one of many small, community-led member

Breaking Barriers. Robin Lin Miller and George Ayala, Oxford University Press. © Oxford University Press 2024.
DOI: 10.1093/oso/9780197647684.003.0001

organizations throughout the world that sexual and gender minority citizens organize and staff to fill the gaping void in their access to humane care. Guy,[3] the human rights activist[4] who recounted Avenir Jeune de L'Ouest's story to me (Robin) during an interview, was deeply disturbed by the conditions his colleagues endured in detention. Three of the men were living with HIV. News accounts of their arrests allude to the men's fragile health.

> Eight days without ART! And we discussed with the policemen. We said "Please! We just want to take the treatment of these guys." They refused. They were sleeping on the floor. On the floor! With just one bucket. The water that they drink and wash, it was, my God, just impossible. Eight days!

Guy shook his head and sucked in his breath. An exhausted, despairing look replaced his ordinarily warm and gentle expression. He continued:

> After this, these guys are broken. Once community members go through this kind of scenario, they are afraid. They are afraid. Even us! Even me! I am afraid. Because I can be there one day, and police can come and take all of us. We are working, but we are always afraid. We are always afraid. Because we don't know.

Guy paused, perhaps imagining the cold cement floor of a jail cell ache in his bones, before telling me another story—of a gay man beaten in his front yard by his cutlass-wielding landlord, the man's possessions strewn in the yard, his neighbors urging on the violence.

It is startling to observe firsthand how profoundly a hostile country environment affects the daily lives of sexual and gender minority people and how immensely difficult it is for sexual and gender minority people to seek necessary health care in such settings. Stories like that of the staff of Avenir Jeune de L'Ouest and of the man brutally attacked by his landlord are hardly rare, especially in countries that criminalize homosexuality. On visits to Cameroon and to other countries that struggle to meet their constitutional ambitions to ensure safe and quality care to all, sexual and gender minority human rights activists told me time and again that it is often preferable and reasonable to wait until one's deathbed before attempting to access sexual health or HIV-focused care. It seems unfathomable that people would rather die than face humiliation and debasement from health care workers. But people learn from what they see around them. By what they see others endure. From the stories like that of the Avenir Jeune de L'Ouest staff who for 8 days were made to share a bucket filled with excrement and urine, sleep huddled on the filth-covered cement floor of a jail cell, drink putrid unpotable water, and do without lifesaving HIV medications all for the crime of trying to fulfill the health needs of LGBT people living with HIV like themselves. Offering HIV-focused care to sexual and gender minority citizens and advocating for their needs in these places requires considerable bravery. But it should not. It is unimaginably dangerous. But it should not be.

This book tells the story of sexual and gender minority activists in eight countries who formed a transnational partnership called Project ACT to break through barriers to HIV health care caused by stigma, discrimination, and violence. In these pages, we describe the genesis of Project ACT and how these partners accelerated change in institutional structures that impede their constituents from claiming their right to care. We share the conditions and practices that shaped their achievements. We reveal, too, the obstacles and defeats they faced along the path to enabling access to affirming health care. We show how they work, day in and day out, in the face of resistance. We also describe the Project ACT evaluation that underlies this book and illustrate how it contributed to the project.

Our purpose in telling this story is twofold. First, we aim to provide our readers with a window into the nature of and challenges inherent in community-led advocacy work to improve access to HIV care in Africa and the Caribbean. Through the voices of local activists and other stakeholders, we extend theoretical understanding of the complexities of community-led advocacy in the context of anti-LGBT and human rights counter-movements. In this book, we set the advocacy work performed by the Project ACT partners within their national political, economic, cultural, and social context. We discuss the importance of allyship to advocacy work, the power dynamics of Global North–Global South development aid and postcolonial politics, and the damaging effects of homophobic and transphobic stigma and discrimination. A very limited number of action research investigations examine community-led advocacy efforts to increase access to HIV care for sexual and gender minority communities in the Global South. We show how LGBT activists, together with their strategically selected allies, contribute to social progress within their country environments, despite immense obstacles, and describe the processes and factors that facilitate their accomplishments.

Our second purpose is to respond to long-standing calls by community psychologists to take readers behind the scenes of community action projects to offer insight on the complexities and challenges of community psychology in action. Addressing structural causes of social injustice is of keen interest to the field, as is investigating community activism. To date, community psychology has not closely examined projects to address human rights concerns or done so in the context of an international effort to secure basic rights for sexual and gender minority citizens. Community psychologists have also not closely explored the unique dynamics of human rights and advocacy evaluation, despite the centrality of advocacy and of evaluation to the field. The setting for our work provides an opportunity to consider the complex tensions that arise in attempting to bring a decolonizing praxis to community psychologists' work. Decolonizing forms of practice may collide with other values such as honoring the sovereign rights of postcolonial independent nations; in this case, these nations practice de jure and de facto political homophobia. In this environment, a professional commitment to ensuring that Indigenous values systems are not undermined by the Global North and that we avoid Western paternalism may clash with the desire to attain equitable ends for sexual and gender minority people. We surface and critically explore these tensions. By illustrating how theories of practice from both community psychology and evaluation work on the ground, we extend practical understanding of the issues and tensions at play when working toward justice and equity[5] with people in their context. We demonstrate why LGBT activists and community-led organizations are critical to the fight to end AIDS in Africa and the Caribbean. We also make the case for transformative evaluations conducted in service of activists' work. We hope that the Project ACT story, and our attempt to make ourselves visible within the telling of that story, prompts readers to reflect on their own positionality, community context, and efforts to contribute to social change.

The Project ACT story is worth telling for many reasons, but it is particularly important at a time when public engagement in the global HIV crisis and funding for HIV initiatives are both in steady decline. Since its discovery, the HIV epidemic has claimed 40.1 million lives.[6] On average, an estimated 4,100 people are newly infected with the virus each day. A majority of these new infections occur among people who are subject to systemic de jure and de facto stigma and discrimination. Understanding how people—including those whose stories we tell—redress the many forms of systematic stigma and discrimination fueling epidemics like HIV is vital. Our book also illustrates what engaged scholarship requires in the context of human rights advocacy. Project ACT provided an all too rare opportunity to embed a scholar within an activist team to document and support the arduous work of enabling access to essential care.

The academic–community partnership George and I forged through this effort was long in the making and rests soundly on the foundation of our nearly 40-year relationship as colleagues. In 2016, after years of working on projects that ticked all the boxes in my university's system of rewards, I had grown deeply discontented at how seldom I experienced a sense of fulfillment in my research, which had gradually become unmoored from the authentic, community-engaged scholarship that served as the bedrock of my career. I felt stuck within the rigid strictures and procedures of a federally funded research portfolio. My impatience to return to projects that felt valuable and community-driven was near the point of boiling over. I had drifted too far from my roots.

I began my career as an evaluator at the Gay Men's Health Crisis (GMHC), the first AIDS-focused advocacy and civil society organization in the world. I worked at GMHC while I was a graduate student finishing my PhD in community psychology at New York University, just as George was completing his PsyD in clinical and community psychology across the river at Rutgers University's Graduate School of Applied and Professional Psychology. GMHC was founded in the living room of the late activist and playwright Larry Kramer to mobilize a response to what was initially termed "gay-related immune deficiency" or GRID. The year I started at GMHC, 1987, the United States Food and Drug Administration approved the first drug for treating HIV—azidothymidine (AZT). AZT came on the market at the astounding cost of $10,000 per year—the equivalent of $26,570 today—just under half the median annual income of $25,990 in 1987 (United States Bureau of the Census, 1989). Condoms had not yet been demonstrated as an effective means of preventing HIV acquisition. President Ronald Reagan enacted a policy prohibiting HIV-infected travelers into the United States. The AIDS Quilt was being prepared for its debut on the National Mall in Washington, DC, comprising 8,288 panels, far smaller than today's 54-ton hand-stitched memorial.

The era during which I worked at GMHC was remarkable for the passionate advocacy work occurring in New York and other hard-hit cities around the globe, advocacy driven by a profound desperation at the indifference of the larger world to the devastation occurring daily in the lives of people affected by HIV. At times, it felt as if we existed on an invisible island, smack dab in the middle of New York City. As the lead evaluator for GMHC's prevention and education units, and later as the founding director of its first agency-wide Department of Evaluation, I conducted multiple internal evaluations of diverse homegrown programs and advocacy efforts to address the rapidly evolving epidemic. Looking back on those 7.5 years, I would argue that my basic training as an evaluator and engaged scholar of the types that community psychology prescribes occurred far less in the classrooms of New York University than it did in GMHC's trenches. GMHC cemented my career trajectory, scholarly interests, and my sensibility toward practicing evaluation and conducting community-engaged research. It led me to create my own approach to evaluation that merges community psychology, action-oriented engaged scholarship, transformative evaluation, and a unified professional identity.

Systematic inquiry and sensemaking are informed by the values and personal histories of the inquirer. Self-location and its examination allow us, and our community partners, to discover the perspectives and experiences that are central to the way we go about our practice, drive our behavior, and guide us in making sense of what we find. It is the basis for reflective practice. Positioning ourselves in relation to others is foundational to building relationships and a central aspect of earning trust; it exposes our commonalities, our differences, and how facets of who we are bring us closer to some and distance us from others.[7] Self-location also prompts awareness of the privileges bestowed on us as engaged scholars. It helps us recognize the limitations of what we see and understand. Truthfully, genuinely, and respectfully locating ourselves in relationships permits us to examine the privilege and power we wield (or lack) as individuals—a dynamic inherent to community-engaged work.

I came to work at GMHC partly because I lived in Fire Island Pines from my birth through my mid-30s. A refuge for gay and bisexual men east of New York City, the Pines and its neighboring community of Cherry Grove were decimated by the early years of the HIV epidemic. I was among many witnesses to the devastation wrought by HIV on the inhabitants of our small 500-house village. Growing up in the Pines and living there part-time well into adulthood profoundly impacted who I have become.[8] I still wake up dreaming I am in my bedroom at 114 Ocean Walk, a room I have not set foot in since 1994. Fire Island Pines is the one place that always recalls my strongest sense of home. The Pines and its people live under my skin. I carry its joys, its freedoms, and its sorrows. Residing in the Pines led directly to the choices I have made throughout my career, beginning with my tenure at GMHC.

I also grew up in the waning years of Jim Crow, a mixed-race child who easily passes as White but who was raised to identify as both Black and European American. This serves as another bridge to my Project ACT colleagues. It plants my feet in a family and community of people who have endured hundreds of years of scorn, prejudice, violence, and degradation. In some sense, I am lucky that my mother's family moved quickly from slavery to the Black middle and professional classes because this enabled my Black ancestors to make privileged experiences available to me that elude many other Black Americans. But their hard-won social position among the Black elite provided them limited protection from overt and de facto discrimination. I know their stories all too well. I also have my own. My appearance makes who I am invisible to others, obscuring from their view a fundamental piece of my identity. I learned to live with a daily uneasiness, which grew from never quite fitting into the majority and from directly confronting assumptions about who I am because of my pale skin and blue eyes. I am uncertain at times if my presence is truly welcome in Black spaces or White spaces. Lightness protects me in some situations, to be sure, but it leaves me vulnerable in others. I am an insider, an outsider, and both all in the same moment. To this day, I experience a visceral physical reaction in my chest, my throat, my arms, my shoulders, and my stomach when others assume I am solely of European descent. When it happens, I feel assaulted, even though I understand it is an easily made mistake. My reaction stems from the erasure of something core to my person. These experiences are not perfect parallels to weathering structural homophobia and transphobia, but they provide me with an experiential basis for empathy and allyship.[9]

When I began to sense that my academic work was no longer serving the gay and bisexual communities that had been so central to my scholarly engagement over decades, I thought of George, whom I had met while working at GMHC. During those early years of the HIV epidemic, George's reputation as a passionate and creative advocate for the rights and needs of gay and bisexual men of color was already well-established. He grew up in government subsidized housing projects on the Lower East Side—a low-income, predominantly Puerto Rican and Black neighborhood at the time—a bridge to his activism. George attended the LaGuardia High School of Music and Art (featured in the movie *Fame*), where he studied visual art. In college, George became enamored with psychology as he began to understand and embrace his queerness—another important bridge to his work. After completing his doctoral coursework in clinical and community psychology, George directed counseling services at New York's Hetrick Martin Institute, the city's largest social service provider for sexual and gender minority youth. Later he became the deputy executive director of the Hispanic AIDS Forum and then moved to California in 1997 for a position at University of California, San Francisco. George went on to assume multiple leadership roles in community-led organizations, on research projects in academic settings, and in public health. George cannot easily be pegged. He is not just a researcher, a civil servant, or a community activist. He is all those things, bringing experiences from each of these domains to his work. At his core, George is a community psychologist with a creative streak, compelled to embed himself in applied settings. In those early years, we often served as community representatives together at scientific think tanks of various kinds. As we argued for—and consistently lost arguments over—the need for a national research agenda that was relevant and responsive to communities most affected by HIV and for support for evaluations of community-led initiatives besides those created by scientists, we quickly realized our worldviews on human sexuality, human rights, and meaningful community engagement in and control over research were strikingly similar. It was perhaps fate, then, that as I sat in the lobby of a hotel in Durban, South Africa in 2016, pondering how I could best recenter my scholarship, George happened to rush through on his way to the espresso bar.

The occasion that brought us to South Africa that summer was the biannual meeting of the International AIDS Society (IAS), the largest global convening of social, behavioral, and clinical scientists, government officials, funders, pharmaceutical companies, activists, and HIV-affected communities in the world. The conference, however, is deceptive. Although it brings these groups together and aspires to unity across the interests they represent, its broad participation hardly signifies collectivism. Rather, the meeting reveals established power dynamics in miniature—the stark imbalance between those who lead society's most important institutions and the diverse community actors who attend the conference hoping to influence how AIDS policies are established and implemented, to shape the questions scientists pursue and the methodologies they use, and to improve the public discourse regarding those who live with or are disproportionately affected by HIV. Ultimately, the meeting is the site of competing and conflicting narratives. Community members who come to this incredibly expensive conference are consigned to its "Global Village," usually a colorful, raucous, steamy unairconditioned tent, or a distant room reminiscent of an airplane hangar. Meanwhile, in the adjacent sleek conference center, scientists, politicians, dignitaries, celebrities, and pharmaceutical representatives rush between sessions and meetings in the air-conditioned chill.

At the time of that meeting in South Africa when I spied George sprinting across the hotel lobby, he had been at the helm of the small yet mighty United States–based human rights advocacy organization, MPact Global Action for Gay Men's Health and Rights, for about a decade. Known simply as MPact, the organization mobilizes and nurtures activist networks in more than 60 countries and advocates at the highest international levels for equitable access to effective HIV prevention, care, treatment, and support services for gay and bisexual men. MPact promotes gay and bisexual men's health and human rights to transnational policy bodies, including the United Nations and the World Health Organization. Cofounded by Australian AIDS activist Don Baxter, MPact began at a time when governments were divesting from community-led HIV responses all over the world, when gay and bisexual men were publicly rendered invisible in forums like the IAS, and when, much like today, cases of HIV infection among gay men were soaring.

Over a 4-year period culminating at the 2006 IAS conference, Don and fellow activists from across five continents—including Aditya Bandopadhyay, Richard Burzynski, Gus Cairns, Robert Carr, Stevie Clayton, Ton Coenen, David Cooper, Carlos García de León, Juan Jacobo Hernandez, Rapeepun Ohm Jommaroeng, Mike Kennedy, Tudor Kovacs, Shivananda Khan, Carlos de Leon, Zhen Li, Samuel Matsikure, Othman Mellouk, John Maxwell, Ken Morrison, Joel Nana, Steave Nemande, Fiona Palmer, Nick Partridge, Midnight Poonkasetwatana, Andy Quan, Leonardo Sánchez, Paul Semugoma, Craig Thompson, and so many more—mobilized and built the global network that would become MPact. During those 4 years, the IAS conference provided a venue for organizing MPact and, ironically, provided an impetus for its necessity.

I was in the Global Village on the day that George took the stage alongside Sir Elton John for a special announcement about a recently established mechanism called the LBGT Fund. Administered by the Elton John AIDS Foundation (EJAF), in partnership with the Joint United Nations Programme on HIV/AIDS (UNAIDS) and the United States President's Emergency Plan for AIDS Relief (PEPFAR), the US$10 million fund would support work with sexual and gender minority communities in Africa via small 2-year grants. MPact was one of two inaugural recipients, funded to lead an 18-month advocacy demonstration project across Africa and the Caribbean to reduce the stigma, discrimination, and violence that impede access to HIV care. It took nearly 2 years for the funding announced at that meeting to make its way to Oakland, California, where MPact is based. During those 2 years, George and I devised a plot to work together. I arrived in Oakland just as the delayed funds did. Although our initial plan was that I would study the role evaluation plays, if any, in MPact's sister networks, George proposed that I instead join the six-person MPact team that would guide the novel demonstration project he had conceived so long ago. This was an ideal vehicle to explore what conducting evaluation in such a context requires, while simultaneously documenting and informing the advocacy work that George, his staff, and our global partners were about to undertake. And, with that, I became a part of the Project ACT team.

We began Project ACT in the spring of 2018 and concluded our work in the spring of 2020, just as the SARS-Cov-2 pandemic upended the world. This book is based on the data I collected throughout those 2 years. The MPact Team and I designed the evaluation collaboratively, with input and participation from our global partners, a process we describe in the section titled "About the Evaluation" toward the end of the book. We drew heavily on principles-focused evaluation[10] (Patton, 2018) and outcome harvesting[11] (Wilson-Grau, 2018; Wilson-Grau & Britt, 2012), both of which are well-suited to the immense challenges and complexities involved in advocacy and human rights evaluation. The data we obtained reflect the work of all our partners. However, due to budgetary constraints we selected four partners to observe intensively. As a result, the experiences and perspectives of our partners from Cameroon, Côte d'Ivoire, Jamaica, and Zimbabwe feature more prominently in the book than those of our other partners.

Our dataset contains interviews I conducted with 112 people who were either in-volved in or closely observed the work. I spoke with several of these people on more than one occasion, including MPact staff and staff in our partner organizations. The data also include field notes of observations I made during my repeated site visits to the four countries noted earlier. Additionally, my field notes include observations of two all-country, learning exchange retreats we held at the start and end of the project; participant observations with MPact staff from the project planning stages through to 8 months beyond the project's conclusion, including notes on interactive activities we engaged in throughout and beyond Project ACT's lifespan. The data also include results of a quantitative survey of partner organizations' staff members, my project diary, and a rich trove of archival documents and photographs. MPact staff, George, and I made sense of emerging findings from these data together and derived impli-cations and lessons on an ongoing basis. Following ethical conventions designed to protect individuals' privacy, coupled with my desire to preserve their relationship to MPact and ensure the confidentiality of their disclosures and identities, I traveled to the countries alone and interacted alone with activists, allies, constituents, and adver-saries as part of the data collection, except when aided by a translator. Besides myself, only trained students working under my supervision at Michigan State University had access to the raw research data for analysis. All other aspects of the work that I describe I performed in close collaboration with George and the other members of MPact's Project ACT team: Omar Baños, Stephen Leonelli, Nadia Rafif, Mohan Sundararaj, Greg Tartaglione, and Johnny Tohme.

Conventionally, evaluators maintain distance from their clients, and purposely so. Even in collaborative evaluations, clients are rarely invited to collaborate with eval-uators in conveying what they learned about their project to the wider world. My relationship with George and the Project ACT team departs from conventional views on how evaluation ought to be practiced. Reflecting our long-standing belief that evaluation ought to engage, nurture, and support community movements for equi-table societies, we instead ground ourselves in the tenets of transformative evaluation (Mertens, 2009) and in community psychology's emancipatory collaborative research practices. Transformative evaluation is among those paradigms that sit closest to community psychology's values and participatory action-oriented methodologies. Both approaches are guided by the principle of social justice. Both aim to elevate the disempowered. Both prioritize the use of engaged systematic inquiry to challenge op-pressive social structures undermining human dignity and wellness. Both, too, are complicated perspectives to employ in the postcolonial settings where Project ACT operated.

We believe that evaluation can, and should, benefit community-led movements. In this vein, George and I are united in our commitment to the same global vision, each playing a distinct, yet mutually supportive, role in its attainment. We share the value of using systematically gathered evidence to identify ways to realize the world we hope to live in. We are both trained social scientists, seasoned in community-engaged action research projects, and traveled in the parts of the world where Project ACT was implemented. We both understand the roles of evaluator and engaged researcher firsthand, just as we both know the daily rhythms of community-led organizations. Yet coauthoring a book comes with challenges. Our workplace imperatives are substantially different. When and how we write are largely dictated by these conditions. We also played distinct roles in the advocacy work we recount. The evaluation focus ultimately anchors the book, so we choose to tell the Project ACT story from that perspective. We write the Project ACT story as a team, engaging with each other on every thought and word, regardless of who first put pen to paper to compose a chapter.[12] Most often, I wrote the first draft. I serve in the role of narrator. In those places where George should serve as primary narrator (e.g., Chapter 3), we indicate he is speaking. We narrate the conclusion together. Throughout the book, true to our belief that evaluation should prioritize individuals' narration of their own experiences, we rely heavily on activists' voices from the participating countries, as well as the voices of MPact staff. Mindful of their privacy and security, we do not use their real names.

Overview of the Book

In Chapter 1, we examine the global context of HIV and set the stage for the work undertaken in Project ACT. We describe why barriers to HIV care for sexual and gender minority people are so intractable and self-perpetuating, with a specific focus on stigma, discrimination, and violence in African and Caribbean contexts. We highlight the challenging postcolonial dynamic that exists among Western nations' imperatives to support human rights for sexual and gender minority people, the role of HIV-focused development aid in supporting these rights, and pushback against human rights claims made in the name of postcolonial independence. In Chapter 2, we argue that the tensions described in Chapter 1 elevate the importance of "movements from within" for realizing human rights goals. We propose that community-led advocacy responses are fundamental to addressing the stigma, discrimination, and violence that impede access to HIV prevention and care. We argue that public health is a strategic entry point to addressing structural causes of HIV risk and human rights violations. The chapter foregrounds tensions and principles of transnational partnerships designed to address access to HIV care for sexual and gender minority people and highlights contemporary work on the often-neglected role of community-led advocacy responses to the epidemic throughout Africa and the Caribbean.

Chapter 3 builds on these previous chapters and describes the origin story of Project ACT. We discuss George's relationship to the work we embarked on together, to MPact, and to the project's transnational partners. We describe the partners' respective national contexts, as these partly explain why they were selected to participate and shaped what was possible to achieve in each setting. Chapter 4 addresses the many complex issues confronting engaged researchers and evaluators who hope to study efforts like Project ACT. We discuss contemporary thinking on how human rights and advocacy evaluation should best proceed, and we highlight the unique ethical and methodological issues that working in the arena of sexual and gender minority human rights presents. We examine the contradictions and tensions that arise when applying existing prescriptions for culturally responsive and socially just evaluation, positioning practice ideals regarding decolonizing processes that respect local cultures and worldviews and honor national sovereignty against the tenets of human rights work and its evaluation. Chapter 4 also introduces my relationship to the work more fully. Finally, the chapter describes the preliminary stages of operationalizing the project's broad vision into actionable advocacy initiatives.

Chapters 5 through 9 concentrate on themes that proved central to Project ACT's implementation, setbacks, and successes. In these chapters we describe the process of nurturing the capacity of activists living in fraught settings, and how we and our partners supported their local constituents to take on advocacy work. Chapter 5 has a particular focus on tactical efforts to reduce internalized stigma, build advocacy capacity, and empower the sexual and gender minority constituencies. In Chapter 6 we address the cultivation of allies. We discuss the motivations for allyship, the role allies played in making advocacy possible, and the challenge of working successfully with allies. Chapter 7 focuses on organizational resilience in the face of adverse events. In every partnership setting, a wide range of challenges emerged: from security threats to political upheaval to disasters to the overwhelming stress of engaging in advocacy against violence and human rights abuses. Some of these challenges were closely tied to the ongoing work, whereas others resulted from increased tensions and uncertainties within wider political, economic, and cultural contexts. Some were merely happenstance. We describe how activists coped with and rebounded from such challenges. Chapter 8 focuses on seeds of change. We detail how the advocacy initiatives progressed, drawing directly on themes of allyship, capacity, resilience, and learning, and examine achievements that were locally meaningful. We also address the limits to what we and our partners accomplished. In Chapter 9, we conclude the book with lessons for supporting community-led work that tries to upend the stigma, discrimination, violence, and criminalization underpinning the HIV epidemic. We highlight the principles of effective partnerships and advocacy practice that guided success, and note how, when these principles were not closely observed, the impact of our collective efforts diminished. We offer policy and practice recommendations for others seeking to remove structural barriers to accessible HIV care within sexual and gender minority communities. We also suggest how to best use evidence when documenting and supporting advocacy. Finally, the Epilogue offers reflections on the importance of community-led advocacy for creating an enabling environment for sexual and gender minority people and the need for evaluation that supports liberatory goals. A detailed account of the evaluation and our collaborative, transformative, evaluation process is provided after the Epilogue. Some readers may prefer to read this description before reading the book's main chapters.

As we write in July of 2023, the COVID-19 pandemic has enflamed the HIV epidemic and set progress to control it backward by as much as a decade.[13] Many of the HIV epidemic's established patterns of inequity are mirrored and reinforced in this new global pandemic. Stigmatized people are hit hardest by COVID-19 and bear the brunt of the public health crisis. Socially marginalized people are most vulnerable to the consequences of lockdowns and their ensuing economic fallout. They experience poor access to the information and resources needed to protect themselves. For them, COVID-19 represents both a socioeconomic and a humanitarian crisis, as they face political scapegoating and escalating abuse. Against this backdrop, learning from community efforts to advance the rights of socially marginalized people in the HIV context can provide a roadmap for relevant responses that reduce social inequities resulting from stigma. Stigma, discrimination, violence, and criminalization place sexual and gender minority people and their health care providers in danger. These human rights abuses undermine our collective ability to solve our most pressing public health crises. Social oppression, in all its forms, imperils our basic humanity. This book honors those activists who place their lives on the line day after day to keep our humanity whole.

PART I

STIGMA AND THE GLOBAL HIV EPIDEMIC

People are afraid, so the work is not easy. I hear difficult stories. I free myself by crying at night.

—Belle, Côte d'Ivoire

The first part of this book, composed of two chapters, investigates the global trends in the HIV landscape that have led to increased vulnerability to HIV infection among gay and bisexual men and transgender people in Africa and the Caribbean. We examine the causes of limited action to address gay and bisexual men's and transgender women's vulnerability and the geopolitical dynamics shaping their vulnerability and neglect. Specifically, we show how stigma, discrimination, and violence targeting gay and bisexual men and transgender women have served as barriers to HIV prevention and care. We explore how formal and de facto efforts to prevent sexual and gender minority community-led organizations from full participation in civil society in Africa and the Caribbean, coupled with the dynamics of development funding, constrain the ability of sexual and gender minority communities to tear down structural barriers that prevent them from accessing affirming HIV prevention and care.

1

We Don't Want to Speak About It

On[1] a steamy July morning in 2012, deep in the bowels of the Washington Convention Center, United States Secretary of State Hillary Rodham Clinton strode onto the stage of the XIX International AIDS Conference. Thunderous applause accompanied her march to the podium. The United States had been denied the right to host the conference for 2 decades, a modest victory for HIV activism. In 1990, AIDS activists from around the world boycotted to protest the International AIDS Society's (IAS) decision to hold the conference in San Francisco. A United States' immigration policy enacted under President Ronald Reagan, a policy steeped in stigma, banned people living with HIV from entering the country, which prevented them from participating in one of the most influential convenings on AIDS in the world. Not until President Obama lifted the discriminatory 22-year ban in 2009 could the conference return to United States' soil. People who inject drugs and sex workers could only participate in the conference remotely, however, as they remain to this day unwelcome.[2]

Most of the audience, and those consigned to watch from abroad, eagerly welcomed Secretary Clinton's appearance because Clinton championed issues of concern to the IAS audience and, in her role as Secretary of State, served as a guarantor of the United States' commitment to an AIDS-free generation. Secretary Clinton's presence also signaled the optimism of the moment, optimism captured in the speech she delivered to the delegates that morning.[3] In her speech, Secretary Clinton trumpeted the incredible biomedical progress that had transformed AIDS from a harrowing death sentence into a chronic yet manageable condition. She applauded the accomplishments of the many highly placed leaders associated with the United States government and those who lead the vital domestic and international institutions that it sponsors. She championed the needs of those women, girls, and orphans who are adversely impacted by HIV throughout the world. Clinton celebrated her State Department's three-pronged combination prevention strategy in Africa and the Caribbean, a strategy that relied on encouraging the uptake of HIV treatment, reducing mother-to-child HIV transmission, and circumcising heterosexual men. She pledged to the audience to eliminate mother-to-child transmission by 2015. She proudly touted the 400,000 circumcisions already performed in Africa, promising that another half a million men and boys would be circumcised in South Africa alone. "If you are not getting excited about this, please raise your hand and I will send someone back to check your pulse," she proclaimed to applause and laughter. Winding toward her conclusion, Clinton called for improved global coordination and greater investments. She urged the assembled world leaders to engage in what she

Breaking Barriers. Robin Lin Miller and George Ayala, Oxford University Press. © Oxford University Press 2024.
DOI: 10.1093/oso/9780197647684.003.0002

termed "difficult conversations," a veiled reference to a disease "transmitted the way that AIDS is" among those at greatest risk. She laid out the work yet to do. She promised to bring AIDS to an end. She brought the crowd to its feet.

Seated in the back row of the darkened auditorium, I (Robin) routinely monitored the methodical tick of the minute hand circling the face of my wristwatch while Secretary Clinton progressed through the key points of her impassioned 34-minute-and-47-second speech. 5 minutes. 9 minutes. 17 minutes. Just after the 25-minute mark, in a single sentence it took her only 15 seconds to utter, Clinton referred to men who have sex with men. Just that once. Even when recalling the first time she viewed the AIDS quilt carpeting the national mall in 1996—a mournful display of more than 8,000 hand-stitched panels that primarily memorialized gay and bisexual men lost to the epidemic—Clinton made no reference to those for whom the panels were stitched. A 34-minute-and-47-second speech. Men who have sex with men: 15 seconds. Transgender people: 0 seconds.

When the speech ended and the auditorium lights rose, I pushed my way through the crowd, overcome by what Clinton had chosen not to say. I headed for the Global Village—the space that best captures the HIV epidemic's true impact and showcases community resistance against its sobering inequities. There, moving past exhibits celebrating the resilience and dignity of the people who Clinton did not name or include on her agenda, the politics of the morning became more maddening for its predictability. Clinton's speech was unsurprising in its emphasis on cisgender women and girls, given her political mission to elevate their unique concerns on many issues, and because of the HIV epidemic's heavily disproportionate impact on women and girls in Southern and Eastern Africa. Her speech was unsurprising in its emphasis on United States government contributions to global problem-solving on HIV, given the extent to which the United States' scientific and financial contributions to the epidemic have been and remain essential. Her speech was unsurprising in its celebration of the latest biomedical advances that address an entrenched, yet preventable, epidemic that has slaughtered millions of people. Her speech was unsurprising in its display of political savvy, its skillful recognition of which issues she might successfully advance with the political dignitaries attending the conference, and which might meet with their vociferous opposition. Her speech, therefore, was unsurprising in its limited emphasis on sexual and gender minority people. Rarely do sexual and gender minority people take center stage in such international forums, except when they storm it to protest their invisibility.[4] Storming the stage is one among many advocacy tactics sexual and gender minority communities have learned they must deploy to be seen, to be heard, and to be meaningfully included in the response to AIDS.

This book tells the story of what happened when a transnational team of human rights–focused sexual and gender minority HIV activists banded together to address obstacles to HIV care enabled by homophobic and transphobic stigma. In this chapter, we describe the global trends in the HIV landscape that set the stage for their collective effort. In the years preceding their joint advocacy, the world witnessed stunning biomedical progress in combating HIV and an unprecedented international commitment to bringing the HIV epidemic under control. The optimism generated by these highly effective biomedical tools coincided with reduced investment in eliminating the obstacles to HIV care that contribute to long-standing inequities among stigmatized populations. Addressing the stigma, discrimination, and violence directed toward gay and bisexual men and transgender women were among the barriers that received limited global attention, except from inside these communities themselves. In this chapter, we discuss how these dynamics shaped these population's vulnerability to HIV, especially the experiences of gay and bisexual men and transgender women in Africa and the Caribbean. We also examine how these dynamics are shaped by factors such as criminalization and colonial and post-colonial influences.

The End of AIDS: A Leaky Pipe Dream

The years immediately before and after Clinton's speech witnessed a remarkable shift in scientific progress toward combating the epidemic. HIV treatment replaced condoms as the global community's most effective form of HIV prevention. Groundbreaking clinical trials demonstrated that antiretroviral therapy, when prescribed quickly after an HIV diagnosis and taken continuously, substantially improves the health of people living with HIV. Scientific studies offered compelling evidence that compliance with an antiretroviral therapy regimen suppresses HIV viral loads to an undetectable point, rendering it impossible for an HIV-infected person to transmit it to others. If nearly every person living with HIV learned their HIV status as soon as possible after their initial infection, received immediate and competent medical care, received antiretroviral therapy, and took it as prescribed, then an AIDS-free generation could be quickly realized.[5] The end of AIDS was in clear sight, or so we were meant to think.

Buoyed by optimism at the promise of these biomedical interventions, the same developments that Clinton hailed in her speech, the global public health community had established an ambitious set of targets by 2014—a fast-track strategy to bring the AIDS epidemic down to a manageable state by 2030. Referred to as the "90-90-90" targets, the fast-track strategy called for its 168 national signatories to ensure that by the end of 2020, 90% of their HIV-infected citizens knew their HIV status, 90% of those individuals received antiretroviral therapy, and 90% of the individuals placed on antiretroviral therapy achieved an undetectable viral load. If each of these targets were met, the annual number of new global infections was projected to drop by 500,000. By 2030, the plan called for these targets to rise to 95%, further reducing the number of new infections per year. Experts and community leaders concurred that success in moving HIV-infected people along this continuum of care—a metaphorical pipeline that moves a person from first learning their HIV status to finally achieving an undetectable and untransmissible viral load in their bloodstream—formed the ideal pathway to ending the epidemic, especially when coupled with initiatives to link high-risk uninfected people to antiretroviral medications as prophylaxis.

At the time, public health experts and community activists were both clearly aware that technical solutions would not be enough. By themselves, manufacturing effective biomedical technologies, expanding HIV testing and clinical services, and improving medication delivery supply chains were still insufficient for pushing the epidemic toward a manageable state. Ensuring that all people pursued HIV testing, and that those who were HIV-infected quickly accessed and sustained their treatment, would require a concerted global effort. In particular, the 2014 plan acknowledged that reaching the goals for 2020 and 2030 meant eliminating the stigma and discrimination that prevent high-risk populations from successfully entering and moving along the continuum of care. Biomedical innovations would simply not result in progress if the fundamental social inequities fueling the epidemic persisted. No one disagreed. Yet, when United States President William Jefferson Clinton took to the stage of the XXII International AIDS Conference in Amsterdam in 2018, the optimism that Secretary Hillary Clinton had expressed just 6 short years earlier was muted at best. By then it was clear the odds of attaining the 2020 targets were not worth the bet (Marsh et al., 2019). As pipelines (and pipe dreams) go, everyone was coming to terms with just how severely and inequitably the continuum of care continued to leak.

An Epidemic of Inequity

By the end of 2017, in the lead-up to the Amsterdam conference, 36.9 million people were living with HIV. An estimated 1.8 million people were newly infected in that year alone; 900,000 died (UNAIDS, 2018).[6] Remarkable progress was being made in addressing the virus's general spread, but in an overwhelming majority of countries, not nearly enough progress to meet the 90-90-90 goals. HIV incidence and AIDS mortality rates both remained too high and their rates of decline simply too gradual (UNAIDS, 2019). By the end of 2018, only 14 countries were on track to reach the targets (ultimately achieving them) (UNAIDS, 2020a). On average, the remaining 154 countries had dramatically improved citizens' access to HIV testing and treatment.[7] But these successes and overall average improvements masked the persistence of stubborn and troubling inequities.[8] In 2017, for example, despite general declines in infections over whole populations, almost half of new infections (47%) came from just five categories of people and their sexual partners—gay, bisexual, and other men who have sex with men; sex workers; transgender people; injection drug users; and the incarcerated (UNAIDS, 2018). By the end of 2018, these groups accounted for more than half of new infections (UNAIDS, 2019). And, by the end of 2019, 62% of new infections (UNAIDS, 2020b).[9] The evidence was indisputable. These five groups and their sexual partners, sometimes called "key populations,"[10] were being left behind. In Europe and Central Asia, the Middle East, North Africa, Western and Central Europe, North America, and Asia and the Pacific, an estimated 96%–99% of new infections occurred in just these groups. In the Caribbean, Latin America, and West and Central Africa, these groups composed 60%–77% of new infections.

As we write, these five groups of people and their sexual partners comprise the largest share of new infections in every region of the world.[11] Consistent with this trend, between 2010 and 2019, new HIV infections increased 25% among gay and bisexual men and 5% among transgender people (UNAIDS, 2020c). Set against a decade of general declines in new infections and mortality rates, these data demonstrated that inequities driven by stigma and discrimination were among the primary obstacles preventing the international community from achieving the 2020 midterm 90-90-90 objectives.[12] Few HIV activists were surprised.

Stigma, Human Rights, and Epidemics

The interplay between stigma and human rights violations offers a useful heuristic framework for explaining the international failure to address the HIV epidemic equitably. It also foreshadows the challenges that must be overcome if the global vision of eliminating the epidemic is to be achieved. The relationship between stigma and human rights is useful, too, for understanding the perspective adopted by many activists: that addressing the HIV epidemic hinges on securing and protecting human rights. The powerful impact of stigma on vulnerability to HIV disease is well known. Writing on stigma 2 decades ago, Aggleton, Parker, and Maluwa observed that AIDS "plays into, and reinforces, existing social inequalities. These include inequalities of wealth, inequalities that make women inferior to men, inequalities of nationality and ethnicity, and inequalities linked to sexuality and different forms of sexual expression" (2003, p. 5). Throughout its 40-year history, the HIV epidemic has been defined by such entrenched inequities, reflected in the disproportionate concentration of new infections in an exceedingly small number of highly stigmatized groups, as well as in women and girls in regions such as Eastern and Southern Africa.

Stigma produces inequities in well-being through a systematic social process of devaluing, in which specific groups of people are designated by other groups as unworthy of fair and respectful treatment (Aggleton et al., 2003). The attributes that lead to stigmatization are not inherently meaningful. They only become meaningful through an active process of social construction, the process by which people come to agree on what constitutes social reality (Link & Phalen, 2001). Increasingly, scholars understand stigma through its role in producing social hierarchies and maintaining a state of powerlessness among the stigmatized. Nonstigmatized people enhance their own power and privilege by conferring stigma onto others. Stigma strips stigmatized people of the agency to make decisions over things for which nonstigmatized people freely exercise their will (Farmer, 2005; Friedman et al., 2021; Link et al., 2018; Parker & Aggleton, 2003). Stigmatized people lose social status because they are viewed as deficient and blameworthy in the eyes of the nonstigmatized; the stigmatized become responsible for the circumstances they endure. Stigma undermines the well-being of stigmatized people by providing nonstigmatized people with reasonable and justified bases for individual, familial, community, and societal acts of discrimination. In essence, stigma provides a rationale for prejudiced behavior. Denying services and entitlements to the stigmatized and treating these individuals in dehumanizing and exclusionary ways is justified based on prejudices born of stigma. Peace scholar Johan Galtung (1969) refers to this phenomenon as structural violence, by which he means the systematic ways in which social structures and institutions kill certain groups of people by preventing them from satisfying their basic needs.

Stigma is enacted at three distinct ecological levels: intrapersonal, interpersonal, and structural (Hatzenbuehler, 2018). Intrapersonal stigma refers to how individuals respond to stigmatization, such as self-loathing or excessive sensitivity to rejection. Interpersonal stigma encompasses acts of microaggression, harassment, victimization, and physical, financial, and emotional violence. Structural stigma or violence encompasses the societal constraints placed on individuals through normative cultural practices and institutional policies (Hatzenbuehler & Link, 2014), such as the criminalization of HIV transmission, exposure, and nondisclosure, as well as the criminalization of same-sex sexual relationships. Stigma's connection to human rights is clear: Structural and interpersonal forms of stigmatization violate individuals' fundamental rights to safety, health, and security, and leave them vulnerable to discriminatory actions. Violating human rights, in turn, reinforces the very structural violence on which such violations are based.

Sexual and Gender Minority Stigma

The principal focus of this book concerns "key populations" who are sexual or gender minorities. Stigmas associated with sexual and gender minority statuses have impeded timely and effective responses to the HIV epidemic since the epidemic's discovery (Altman et al., 2012). Sexual and gender minority populations do not necessarily comprise a cohesive group, imbued with a well-articulated and shared system of values (Miller, 2018). Sexual and gender minority people are diverse in their culture, nationality, age, race, ethnicity, class, disability status, romantic and emotional attraction, sexual identity, and gender identity and expression. There may be no outwardly obvious connection among members of sexual and gender minority populations, particularly in settings that openly discourage these populations from forming organized, cohesive communities. Nonetheless, sexual and gender minority people share in their stigmatization, which often manifests as structural violence, and in the consequential need for support from others with these same shared experiences. Pervasive stigma against sexual and gender minority people also fuels observed disparities in their health and well-being (Valdesseri et al., 2019). Stigma constrains the opportunities available to sexual and gender minority people for achieving optimum health outcomes by permitting overt and legalized discrimination against them, providing a normative basis for their ill treatment, and by fostering their social isolation. Stigma (and the structural violence it fuels) manifests in where sexual and gender minority people can safely live, how they may be treated when they engage with local institutions, and the amount of funding that societies spend on providing access to nondiscriminatory and affirming health care. Through the regulation and distribution of opportunity and punishment, therefore, stigma significantly affects sexual and gender minority individuals' social and material experiences.

Stigma's role in producing negative health outcomes for sexual and gender minority people also includes the mental stress incurred by enduring and anticipating its manifestations. Stigma produces health disparities through stress-associated cognitive, behavioral, and physiological mechanisms (Meyer, 2003; Pachankis & Lick, 2018). Specifically, research among sexual and gender minorities finds that cognitive and emotional responses to stigma include hypervigilant anxiety in anticipation of stigma and rejection; low self-regard; loneliness; depression; and rumination. Behavioral processes triggered by stigma include concealment of identity, including from health care providers; avoidance of health services; and excess risk-taking resulting in harm to oneself and others (e.g., substance abuse, tobacco use). Physiological responses to chronic stress include disruptions to proper coordination among the hypothalamus, pituitary gland, and adrenal gland; weakened immune function; accelerated cellular aging; and exaggerated cardiovascular reactivity. In simple terms, the sheer stress of enduring ongoing stigma undermines a person's mental and physical health.

Until recently, sexual and gender minority people were rarely the focus of empirical investigations examining how stigmatizing processes undermine their well-being or overall health (Coulter et al., 2014; Institute of Medicine Committee on Lesbian, Gay, Bisexual, and Transgender Health Issues and Research Gaps and Opportunities, 2011). The available evidence, principally from the United States and Western Europe, indicates that sexual and gender minority populations suffer from an array of health concerns, and at rates far higher than those observed in the general population. Research also shows that these health concerns are clearly shaped by the cognitive, behavioral, and physiological reactions to interpersonal and structural stigma (Meyer, 2003). Entrenched disparities, some of which have reached epidemic levels, have been documented across the many different subgroups comprising sexual and gender minority populations. These disparities appear across the lifespan, in the domains of infectious disease, chronic noninfectious disease, psychological illness, and social pathology, most notably victimization from multiple forms of individual and structural violence (see, for example, Austin et al., 2016; Diaz et al., 2001; Frederiksen et al., 2017; Hatzenbuehler, 2017; Hatzenbuehler & Pachankis, 2016; Hatzenbuehler et al., 2014; Hughes et al., 2011; Kosciw et al., 2015; Meyer et al., 2017; Miller, 2018; Mustanski et al., 2016). Studies conducted throughout the world now illustrate stigma's exponential impact when multiple stigmas intersect, documenting higher rates of traumatic experiences among people of color, those whose gender expression is perceived as nonconforming, and those who are disadvantaged economically (Santos et al., 2021). Studies from throughout the world also link structural sexual minority stigma to individuals' discomfort in interacting with primary care providers, especially regarding discussions of sex and sexual health. Structural stigma is linked to the denial of health care services and the provision of substandard care. Discrimination in the provision of health care, including mental health care, is also associated with delayed access to care. These delays mean diseases are often too severely advanced to avoid permanent disability or premature mortality (Logie et al., 2020).

Cross-national studies clearly illustrate the pernicious effect of stigma on sexual and gender minority people's well-being. Across the globe, gay, bisexual, and other men who have sex with men report persistent stigma and discrimination among health care providers when attempting to access HIV services. Such surveys of gay and bisexual cisgender men and transgender people establish clear links among stigma, criminalization, and access to HIV services. Stigma is greater in countries that criminalize sex between men, which, in turn, results in the lower use of HIV services compared to noncriminalizing countries (Arreola et al., 2015; Ayala & Santos, 2016; Ayala et al., 2018; Santos et al., 2017). This relationship between criminalization and lower service use thus results in a substantially higher HIV prevalence in such countries (UNAIDS, 2021a, 2021b).

Stigma, Sexual and Gender Minority Human Rights, and HIV in Africa and the Caribbean

International research on these issues is limited in some global regions and national contexts because criminalization and extreme stigma both discourage research and create tremendous obstacles to conducting it well. Consequently, research on how stigma affects sexual and gender minority people in sub-Saharan Africa and the Caribbean has been slow to accumulate (Chakrapani, 2021; Fitzgerald-Husek et al., 2017). Available evidence affirms that sexual and gender minorities are highly vulnerable to almost insurmountable stigma-induced challenges and to human rights violations. These include blackmail; state-based and police harassment; food and financial insecurity; unemployment; homelessness; and physical, sexual, financial, and emotional violence. These challenges, in turn, are linked to heightened HIV risk (Logie et al., 2018, 2019; Rodriguez-Hart et al., 2017).

In many national contexts, there are severe social and legal penalties for engaging in same-sex sexual relationships or expressing a sexual or gender minority identity. In 2020, there were 68 countries around the world, from Jamaica to Saudi Arabia to Nigeria, where engaging in consensual same-sex sexual behavior among males was punishable under the law, with sanctioned punishments including castration, torture, mandatory decades-long imprisonment, and death.[13] In 57 countries, transgender people were similarly criminalized. Transgender people are also vulnerable to same-sex criminalization laws through the process of misgendering.[14] In such hostile contexts, claiming a sexual and gender minority identity may be conditioned by intense fear, especially in places where laws require citizens to report sexual and gender minorities to the authorities. Exercising one's right to everyday opportunities may be difficult, if not impossible. HIV transmission, exposure, and nondisclosure are also criminalized in 89 countries, including several states in the United States (UNAIDS,

2021a). Laws that criminalize HIV transmission, exposure, and nondisclosure can sometimes operate as proxies for homophobic structural violence directed at sexual and gender minority people.[15] As of July 2020, 42 of the countries that criminalize homosexuality were located within Africa and the Caribbean (Human Rights Watch, 2020; International Lesbian, Gay, Bisexual, Trans, and Intersex Association, 2021). Projections also suggest we are in great danger of failing to meet global targets for the epidemic's end within the African diaspora, due in part to criminalization and widespread stigmatization.[16]

In 2020, global regions with the highest adult prevalence of HIV infection were Eastern and Southern Africa (6.7%), West and Central Africa (1.4%), and the Caribbean (1.1%). Four Caribbean countries accounted for roughly 90% of HIV cases in that region—Cuba, the Dominican Republic, Haiti, and Jamaica. Historically, Africa and the Caribbean were thought to differ in that in sub-Saharan Africa, the epidemic continues to be viewed as a "generalized epidemic," whereas in the Caribbean it is understood to be concentrated in "key populations," the vulnerable groups to which we referred earlier: gay, bisexual, and other men who have sex with men; people who inject drugs; sex workers; and transgender people. In Jamaica, for example, gay and bisexual men have an estimated HIV prevalence of roughly 28%–31%, and transgender women of 25%–52% (Figueroa et al., 2013, 2015; Logie et al., 2016). Characterizations of a generalized sub-Saharan African epidemic have been contested as inaccurate, however, given long-standing evidence of concentrated and unaddressed subepidemics in certain populations. Although women and girls represent the highest absolute number of new HIV infections in Eastern and Southern Africa, people who use drugs, sex workers, prisoners, men who have sex with men, and transgender women shoulder a disproportionate HIV disease burden in Eastern and Southern Africa, as they do everywhere.[17] HIV prevalence and incidence in "key population" groups are disproportionately high relative to their population size. For instance, recent studies and systematic reviews suggest that the prevalence of HIV among sexual minority men in sub-Saharan Africa is roughly five times that of other males (Hessou et al., 2019; Poteat et al., 2017), a figure that many believe is underestimated, given limited epidemiologic data on the population.

Success in curtailing infections among sexual and gender minority people in sub-Saharan Africa and the Caribbean is limited, with progress toward achieving the mid-term 90-90-90 targets abysmal. When Project ACT began, only 24% of sexual minority men living with HIV in sub-Saharan Africa were estimated to be on antiretroviral therapy (Stannah et al., 2019). Of those receiving treatment, only 25% attained viral suppression. Available data showed extraordinarily high rates of HIV infection, as well as poor engagement along the treatment cascade (Smith et al., 2021). The combination of criminalization and entrenched social stigmatization in Africa and the Caribbean also manifested in these groups' HIV-related needs receiving minimal attention. In the World Health Organization's 2018 review of 45 National AIDS Strategic Plans in Africa, only 10 mentioned transgender people, of which only four outlined limited programming (World Health Organization, 2018).

Most plans mentioned sexual minority men, but few outlined specific programs for enabling access to antiretroviral therapy or discussed the use of strategies such as community-based testing. Epidemiologic data about men who have sex with men and transgender people in the National AIDS Plans were often limited to reports of HIV prevalence. Even so, just half of all plans in the 2018 review reported HIV prevalence among sexual minority men, and only one plan reported prevalence among transgender people. Although plans referenced the World Health Organization recommended package of interventions for people designated as members of "key populations," structural interventions—including activities to remove barriers to service access and use—were seldom included. Few national plans recommend the review of laws and practices criminalizing sex between men, despite the World Health Organization's recommendation to do so. Few mentioned the need to sensitize health care providers as a strategy for addressing stigma and discrimination in the health care field, despite research indicating that poor treatment by health care workers impedes access (Gyamerah et al., 2020; Ross et al., 2021). A contemporary review of National AIDS Plans documents revealed that few plans in Eastern and Southern Africa included indicators or activities, and none include budgetary allocations to address HIV among transgender people (Castellanos et al., 2022). The structural impediments to accessing affirming HIV care are immense in these regions and speak to the enormity and importance of concerted advocacy efforts to remove them.

Colonial Influence on Sexual and Gender Minority Human Rights: Past and Present

The human rights of sexual and gender minorities are a salient aspect of global politics, including throughout the African diaspora, where homophobia and transphobia exist within a complex colonial past and a present postcolonial dynamic (Aldrich, 2003; Epprecht, 2008, 2010, 2012; McKay, 2016; Semugoma et al., 2012). Although many Western countries share the conviction that human rights are universal and should extend to sexual and gender minority people, their commitment to promoting the human rights of sexual and gender minority people has sown sharp divisions that play out in the context of contemporary development aid (Currier & Cruz, 2014; Onapajo & Isike, 2016). Development aid is viewed by some governments as a means by which North America and Western Europe bludgeon their countries toward a more accepting view of sexual and gender minority human rights. Some scholars of the African diaspora suggest that the claim of universal human rights frames Western liberal ideas regarding sexual and gender minority people as significantly more enlightened than the rest of the world's ideas, echoing the patronizing colonial attempts to "civilize" Africa and Africans (Rao, 2014). In this discourse, homosexuality is a colonial import—imposed upon nations in Africa, the Caribbean, and elsewhere, via the assertion of Western (White European) superior values and beliefs. However, the public moral codes condemning homosexuality in Africa and the Caribbean are colonial in their language and origins (Altman et al., 2012), leading to the counter-assertion that what Western colonial powers imposed on Africa, the Caribbean, and other colonized regions was not homosexuality, but their own homophobia. As Rao (2014) cautions, as far as sexual and gender minority rights are concerned, no region of the world has escaped from ugly and dehumanizing behavior.

Britain provides an obvious case in point, as it has had a large and enduring legal impact on its former colonies (Human Rights Watch, 2008). Britain imposed a legal framework on its colonies, grounded in Judeo-Christian beliefs and its own Offences Against the Person Act of 1828, which built on Britain's Buggery Act of 1553. This act, among other things, criminalized sodomy and laid the foundation for present-day statutes criminalizing sex between men in Britain's former colonies. Jamaica's criminalization code, for instance, dates to 1864 during the period of British colonial rule. Although the British began the process of dismantling its criminalization law in 1967, many British colonies gained independence prior to that point. Although some former colonies, such as India, have since overturned the criminalization laws that were part of its colonial inheritance, many others have retained those laws and, in some cases, sought to strengthen them after independence. Other colonial powers also imported homophobia in the form of criminalization. France, although it decriminalized same-sex sexual relations in 1971, imposed criminalization on its colonies as a means of social control of colonized peoples. The legacy of French colonial laws remains active in Francophone countries, including those routinely cited for egregious violations of sexual and gender minority human rights, such as Cameroon.

Despite their historical role in shaping contemporary beliefs on homosexuality in regions such as Africa and the Caribbean, Western nations have increasingly used sexual and gender minority human rights as a condition of their development aid (Namwase et al., 2017). African political leaders have pushed back especially hard against these contingencies, viewing them as attempts at colonial domination. Among the more famous examples of open defiance of the West's attempt to promote sexual and gender minority human rights was a 2011 radio address by Robert Mugabe. Responding to David Cameron's conditioning of British foreign aid on Zimbabwean tolerance of homosexuality, Mugabe asserted that homosexuals are "worse than pigs and dogs" (United Press International, November 25, 2011). The president of Gambia made a similar rebuff in 2014, equating defense of his nation's sovereignty with the unwavering and vehement rejection of sexual and gender minority human rights:

> We will fight these vermin called homosexuals or gays the same way we are fighting malaria-causing mosquitoes, if not more aggressively.... We will therefore not accept any friendship, aid or any other gesture that is conditional on accepting homosexuals or LGBT as they are now baptized by the powers that promote them. (Reuters Staff, February 8, 2014)

Scholars often refer to these public statements by politicians as forms of political homophobia, the vehement expression of anti-gay sentiments to serve an ulterior political purpose (Currier, 2019). Political homophobia, as scholars point out, is a strategy used by leaders and political parties to establish their authority. It can be used to assess political support, to deflect attention from issues on which politicians are vulnerable, or to scapegoat and redirect blame for issues of national concern. In 2021, for instance, ultraconservative politicians in Senegal used homophobic rhetoric to test their election viability and whether they could unify disparate conservative political and religious groups around an anti-gay agenda. A well-documented consequence of these vitriolic positions is socially sanctioned violence against sexual and gender minority people (Awondo et al., 2012; Müller et al., 2021; White & Carr, 2005). Religious perspectives originating in Judeo-Christian, Muslim, and Evangelical traditions also play a critical role in the maintenance of homophobic social positions and public discourse (Currier & Cruz, 2014: Kaoma, 2016).

Marc Epprecht, a renowned scholar of homosexuality and homophobia in Africa, points to the jarring contradictions between publicly expressed intolerance of homosexuality, including equating anti–gay rights positions with national loyalty, and Africans' day-to-day indifference to what one does behind a closed door. The public-private distinction and the willingness to tolerate sexual behaviors away from the public eye are perceived as one reason why Western-styled advocacies run afoul of local norms. As Guy, the Cameroonian activist, explained when I visited him in 2019, public acknowledgment of sexuality and political homophobias are on a collision course in his country:

> It is not only for homosexuality issues. In Cameroon, when you do your thing in your room, no problem. But when you want to march. You want to make some modification of our rights. Because what I see now with political crises,[18] people are not allowed even to put their fingers outside. When you try, they will cut.

As he spoke, Guy pointed his right index finger at me and used his left hand as an imaginary cleaver severing the finger from the rest of his hand. Guy offered an example of general intolerance of public sexuality, noting that when the Cameroonian Ministry of Education recently attempted to add a module on sexual health to the standard high school textbook, there was broad public outcry:

> Oh my God, Robin, it was like boom! Nobody wanted to see that. Nobody. Nobody. Even from a gay man, I was surprised. Nobody wanted [it]. We don't want to think about it. We don't want to speak about it.

Tarone, a legal scholar I interviewed in Jamaica in 2018, characterized the dynamic in his country similarly, as he responded to my question about public opinion regarding sexual and gender diversity: "But it's fine if they are gay and keep it to themselves and don't bring it out into public. But when it comes to the actual human rights of living, it becomes tricky." These norms drive the common perceptions that Africa and the Caribbean simply lack sexual and gender minority people and lead to the oversimplified belief that countries in these regions are uniformly more homophobic than the rest of the "civilized world" (Awondo et al., 2012). Scholars caution that the historical trajectory and dynamics of political homophobia may differ substantially from one nation to the next, despite the results for sexual and minority citizens being largely the same (Bertolt, 2019).

Foreign Aid Dependence

In their attempts to address their HIV epidemics, low- and middle-income countries throughout the African diaspora are highly dependent on development aid (UNAIDS, 2020d; Wamai, 2014). During the 2010s, HIV investments from major global donors shifted toward Africa and decreased elsewhere. Simultaneously, however, worldwide investment in HIV declined. Countries receiving funds from large international donors, especially middle-income countries, faced mounting pressure to invest their own domestic resources in managing their national epidemics. For example, Global Fund investment in Jamaica's HIV response declined by roughly 48% in just a few years, from $19.1 million in the 2014–2016 funding cycle to $9.9 million in the 2017–2019 funding cycle, forcing the Jamaican government to find alternative funding for antiretroviral therapy. Between 2010 and 2019, the proportion of investment in national AIDS programs shifted toward an increased share of domestic funding. However, beginning in 2017, domestic investment started to shrink, with a disproportionate impact on services for sexual minority men and transgender people. In hard-hit regions of Africa, domestic investment in programming declined by 12%–14% (UNAIDS, 2020a, 2020d).

Despite international efforts aimed at aligning funds with the rights and needs of sexual and gender minority communities, and in support of community-led responses,[19] minimal spending is ultimately devoted to these communities—a circumstance that shrinking resources is likely to exacerbate (Avert, 2020). One study suggested that although gay and bisexual men accounted for roughly 20% of new global HIV infections between 2016 and 2018, funding to address their needs comprised 1% of the US$57 billion donors directed at the epidemic during those years (AidsFonds, 2020). In the face of a global decline in HIV funding, support for programming directed at "key populations" is especially endangered, as these programs rely heavily on international sources of support within national AIDS portfolios.

Containing HIV through international development resources points to another complicating postcolonial dynamic, one that recognizes how international development aid is often an instrument of diplomacy and a means to advance the political interests of donor countries. Tensions thus exist between public health and human rights imperatives, on the one hand, and neoliberal (neocolonial) policies designed to maintain and expand exploitable markets, on the other. China, for example, has heavily invested in Africa and the Caribbean for 40 years, expanding markets in the region, but it does not place human rights contingencies on its development funding or infrastructure investments. Understood in this context, therefore, a focus on general population HIV responses in Africa and the Caribbean makes sense; the United States and other Western donors have a geopolitical interest in slowing China's economic expansion in these regions, but their investments come with requirements that many African and Caribbean politicians find unpalatable.

Global funding patterns also create a conundrum for sexual and gender minority human rights activists throughout the African diaspora, as they must often position their work at the intersection of HIV and public health. HIV dominates the funding landscape, a topic we discuss in Chapter 2, which naturally incentivizes a combined HIV and a sexual and gender minority emphasis. But it is also exceedingly difficult for sexual and gender minority-led organizations to legally register as LGBT-focused human rights organizations in hostile national contexts. Legal registration is important because it allows community-led organizations to open bank accounts and receive domestic and foreign assistance. In some countries, therefore, the only path to legal recognition available to sexual and gender minority human rights organizations is to register as an HIV organization (or a mainstream human rights organization). However, this burdens sexual and gender minority human rights–focused community-led organizations with the often-onerous demands of the HIV international donor community or dilutes their focus on sexual and gender minority rights (Currier & Cruz, 2014).

Community-led organizations are critical to the global HIV response and to advancing sexual and gender minority human rights. Both causes deserve a dedicated focus. Community-led HIV responses have multiple advantages over public and private sector services. These include improved HIV prevention, care, and clinical outcomes when compared with responses led by clinics or large governmental organizations. Community-led responses are also associated with improvements in service availability and coverage, linkage to and use of care, care acceptability, patient retention, and service coordination and quality (Argento et al., 2016; Ayala et al., 2021; Baptiste et al., 2020; Denison et al., 2020; Fox et al., 2019; Janamnuaysook et al., 2022; Kerrigan et al., 2015; Nachega et al., 2016; Strömdahl et al., 2019; Suthar et al., 2013; Yang et al., 2020). Funder-imposed programmatic expectations, however, may focus organizational efforts too narrowly on HIV prevention and clinical outcomes. Doing so risks deflecting programing attention away from dismantling the structural causes of discrimination (Currier & McKay, 2017) and addressing other pressing needs that result from stigma and inadequate human rights protections. Activists may be forced to rely on HIV as the entry point, sometimes the only entry point, for combating structural violence and elevating human rights concerns. Offering HIV services and programs, and other public health services, may be the only available route for facilitating collaboration among entities with stakes in public health, both those within and outside government, in addition to mobilizing international aid and transnational activist networks. In many diasporic settings, therefore, HIV and public health represent a safer entry point for organizations, offering some security from governmental backlash that a direct focus on human rights might generate (Awondo et al., 2012;

Epprecht, 2012). However, as we saw with AJO's staff experience in the Introduction, this strategy is by no means perfect.

Conclusion

The biomedicalization of HIV prevention and treatment paradoxically draws attention away from the human rights considerations facing sexual and gender minority communities—considerations that bear directly on their access to lifesaving medical advances. Although heralded as a hard-fought win by activists, HIV responses that are singularly focused on biomedical interventions overlook stigma, discrimination, criminalization, and other social and structural drivers of the epidemic (Aggleton & Parker, 2015). While empowering medical professionals, biomedicalization may confine those people living with, or affected by, HIV—including sexual minority and transgender people—to narrowly defined roles, such as outreach workers, peer educators, or community advisory group members. This undermines community members' decision-making and financial capacity, and further entrenches power among those primarily nonstigmatized people who tend to determine what services and programs are needed (rather than those stigmatized people who use them). Ironically, research on stigma suggests that community empowerment, as well as structural strategies to disrupt anticipated and enacted stigma, are key to its reduction (Dunbar et al., 2020). These strategies include questioning and challenging power inequities, fostering the development of community-led movements, enfranchising sexual and gender minority people's civic participation, advocating to secure sexual and gender minority people's fundamental human rights, and pressuring for access to affirming, high-quality HIV care—all topics we will turn to in Chapter 2.

Although HIV-related work may provide a necessary cover for advancing human rights, the notion that health is a human right itself remains contested. In this context, offering rights-based HIV services to gay and bisexual men and transgender people becomes a dangerous proposition (Epprecht, 2012). Community-led organizations and clinics serving gay and bisexual men and transgender women are routinely vandalized (Beck et al., 2015; Semugoma et al., 2012). Their workers' lives are put at risk simply by attempting to provide the most basic HIV care. Just a year after Secretary Clinton's 2012 speech, an incredibly violent summer in Cameroon led to the suspension of services at four agencies, and to the brutal murder of Eric Lembembe, the newly named executive director of CAMFAIDS, a leading HIV/AIDS nongovernment organization in Yaoundé, the capital city. Lembembe's murder was preceded by a rash of attacks that rocked Cameroon's sexual and gender minority communities. Offices were ransacked and set ablaze. Defenders of sexual and gender minority human rights, as well as HIV service providers and their families, received death threats. Events reached their peak when Lembembe's body was discovered in his home, his feet and hands bound, his feet and neck broken, and his face, hands, and feet scorched with an iron. His murder serves as another gruesome reminder of our collective failure to center the rights of sexual and gender minority people in the global fight against HIV.

Back in July 2012, seated in the cool darkness of the packed Washington Convention Center, with currents of steam rising from the sidewalks in the muggy heat outside, Secretary Clinton's remarks struck me as profoundly troubling. Positioned at the helm of the United States President's Emergency Plan for AIDS Relief (PEPFAR), the largest bilateral funder of the global HIV response, Clinton outlined three strategies to secure her vision. Her list emphasized strategies that were not pertinent to gay and bisexual men and transgender women. It excluded proven strategies for preventing HIV infection among them. It sidestepped the critical roles that stigma and human rights violations play in preventing access to HIV prevention and care, stigmas that drive the burden of HIV onto gay and bisexual men, transgender women, and other "key populations." It frustrated me, as it frustrated George, to no end. If we do not truly embrace a human rights approach that simultaneously invests in sexual and gender minority health, and community-led programming and advocacy, the AIDS-free generation that Secretary Clinton asked us to imagine that morning will remain a pipe dream.

2

Our Power Is Believing in a Better Life Tomorrow

Ghana's Parliament heard its first reading of the "Promotion of Proper Human Sexual Rights and Ghanian Family Values Bill" on August 2, 2021. If successfully passed, the bill will dramatically stiffen Ghana's same-sex criminalization law (Paquette, 2021; Reid, 2021; Rights Africa, 2021). The bill is terrifying for its malevolence. The bill lengthens the maximum prison term for engaging in same-sex sexual activity from 3 to 5 years. It newly prohibits oral and anal sex in all sexual partnerships. It endorses the widely debunked practice of "conversion" therapy.[1] But the bill's most jarring and invidious provisions specify imprisonment of those who advocate for or concern themselves with the rights of sexual and gender minority people in all forms, including conducting academic research, donating funds, making affirming statements on social and in other media, and offering specialized human and social services. If convicted of any type of support or advocacy, people may serve prison terms of up to 10 years.

Despite international pressure to stop the bill from progressing and challenges to its constitutionality, the bill was referred to the Parliament's Constitution and Legal Affairs Committee for review, a preliminary step toward its ultimate enactment into law. Indeed, news accounts suggest the bill has sufficient support within Parliament and among Ghanaian citizens to become law, despite its deadly implications for sexual and gender minority citizens and their allies, its dramatic erosion of Ghanaian democracy and its civil society protections, and its potential to derail the country's HIV response. Behavioral surveillance data for Ghana in 2017 estimated the HIV infection rate for gay and bisexual men at 18%, compared to a rate of roughly 1% among the general population of adult males (UNAIDS, 2021c). Sending the community further underground and cutting off their access to health resources can only increase this disparity. The bill's mere consideration has fueled widespread violence and harassment of sexual and gender minority citizens throughout the country.[2]

The Ghanian bill is not an anomalous attempt to cripple the segments of civil society that advocate on human rights issues concerning sexuality and gender and those that offer LGBT-focused services, including HIV care. Nor did it emerge in a vacuum.[3] This bill, and the events leading up to its drafting, reflect long-standing divisions over the human rights of sexual and gender minority people, divisions that are not peculiar to Ghana. The bill's authors and its secular and faith-based anti-rights champions frame the bill's provisions as necessary to protect Ghana's national

Breaking Barriers. Robin Lin Miller and George Ayala, Oxford University Press. © Oxford University Press 2024.
DOI: 10.1093/oso/9780197647684.003.0003

values and moral character. Portraying sexual and gender minority people as alien to a country's cultural value system is a discursive strategy routinely invoked by conservative Christian, Evangelical, and Muslim groups to prevent LGBT rights–based movements from progressing the world over.[4] Scholars suggest the Christianization of Africa transformed African perceptions of same-sex sexuality from natural to vile, and it set the stage for just this kind of preemptive use of religious ideology to obstruct sexual and gender rights-based movements (Currier & Cruz, 2014; Kaoma, 2016). Framing human rights activists as antinationalist is a common tactic employed to discredit them (Pousadela & Perera, 2021). Challenging their patriotism and branding them as a national threat can deflect activists' attention from addressing matters of policy and practice. It forces activists to focus their attention on preserving their credibility, reputation, constituencies, and public bases of support. As Gutman notes (2001), claims to nationalism, galvanizing though they may prove to be, are far from the same as defending rights to collective self-determination. Nor is nationalism akin to protecting the right of citizens to live free from cruelty, oppression, and degradation. The Ghanian bill illustrates her point.

In this chapter, we situate the work of sexual and gender minority community-led organizations, including our Project ACT partners, and their human rights activism in geopolitical context. We describe the formal and de facto mechanisms that prevent sexual and gender minority community-led organizations and their constituencies from full participation in civil society. We outline how this exclusion obstructs efforts to promote sexual and gender minority human rights, protect sexual and gender minority citizens' health and well-being, and bring an end to the HIV epidemic. We also consider how the dynamics of development funding and international partnerships impact on the ability of sexual and gender minority communities to pursue local advocacy priorities. We extend our argument that a focus on HIV and public health may provide a rare strategic entry point for civic engagement to apply pressure for social change. By addressing the stigma, discrimination, and violence that serve as structural barriers to HIV care and that elevate HIV risk, community-led organizations can further the achievement of human rights goals. They can also reverse the processes through which stigma robs sexual and gender minority people of political, social, and economic agency.

Criminalizing Advocacy and Activists Matters

That Ghana might pursue a tactic common to autocratic regimes is alarming, given its heralded position as an exemplar of democracy in West Africa. Criminalizing sexual and gender minority human rights activists, their organizations, and their allies disables a critical tool for advancing equitable responses to the HIV epidemic: ensuring the opportunity that all people affected by HIV are heard, have access to humane care without fear of discrimination and maltreatment, and that their perspectives are considered on decisions that may affect them. The global contributions of activists to addressing the HIV epidemic are indisputable. Activists focused the world's attention on the discrimination, neglect, and abuse of human rights that characterized the earliest years of the epidemic in an unprecedented fashion (Enoch & Piot, 2017; France, 2016; Lorway, 2017; Schulman, 2021; Trapence et al., 2012). The many advances to which HIV activists have made notable contributions include lowering of AIDS drug prices, adding antiretroviral medications to the international list of essential medicines, improving mechanisms for humane access to treatments, revising national AIDS policies and strategic plans to better serve people affected by HIV, articulating patient rights charters, and pushing for the establishment of the largest global providers of funds to combat the HIV epidemic—the Global Fund to Fight AIDS, Tuberculosis, and Malaria (The Global Fund) and the United States President's Emergency Plan for AIDS Relief (PEPFAR) (Ooms & Hammonds, 2018). Activists were essential to the creation of innovative solutions to slow the spread of the epidemic, including the development of syringe exchange programs, the refinement of harm reduction principles to guide effective intervention for people who use drugs, and the introduction of the U = U campaign (Undetectable equals Untransmittable). U = U underscores the importance of antiretroviral medications, when used as prescribed, for treatment and prophylaxis to prevent HIV.[5]

Many perceive that the activism that led to better management of the HIV epidemic waned in the wake of an increasingly biomedicalized HIV response (Chapter 1), alarming those who recognize that community activists are often best positioned to observe the ill effects of stigma, discrimination, and violence locally and bring these to the table for public examination. Premature declarations that the end of AIDS was in sight (Chapter 1), coupled with AIDS fatigue from a more than 40-year effort to combat the epidemic, have also contributed to declining financial support for activists and rights-based, community-led advocacy (Bekker et al., 2018; Kenworthy et al., 2018). Although these global trends are troubling, the challenges to AIDS activists also stem from their formal and de facto exclusion from participating in civil society in areas of the world hardest hit by the epidemic. Strengthening sexual and gender minority civil society participation to secure their right to access HIV prevention, testing, and treatment free of stigma, discrimination, and violence is a vital component of completing the project to end AIDS everywhere. Activists still have critical work to do.

The Role of Civil Society in the Pursuit of Sexual and Gender Minority Rights to Affirming HIV Care

Although the term "civil society" has been roundly critiqued for its Eurocentric and colonial origins (Daniel & Neubert, 2019; Glasius, 2010) and is far from perfect in its realized forms, it is considered a vital organ of democratic forms of governance. Civil society embodies the public arena of peaceful and open deliberation on matters of public interest. Theoretical hallmarks of functioning civil societies include openness to considering multiple perspectives and welcoming of debate on how best to advance the public good. In its utopian and seldom realized ideal, civil society exemplifies a public life in which citizens are free to voice their needs, interests, and concerns openly and without fear of reprisal. Civil society offers citizens a means to hold their leaders to account for meeting basic subsistence needs, supporting human agency, and ensuring freedom from structural violence (Chapter 1) in all its forms. Citizens may solve their conflicts without resorting to violence or repression. They can act together to prevent their governments and other powerful social actors from pursuing arbitrary action.

The aspirational notion of civil society closely aligns with normative aims of justice and equality, and it ties directly to the task of securing human rights. Healthy civil societies provide the prerequisite conditions for successful pursuit and attainment of human rights. In civil societies that operate effectively, people view one another as equals who share similar stakes in their common society. Given the same stakes, people must act with a commitment to ensuring the realization of rights and entitlements for everyone, not just themselves, or their tribes, or their communities of identity. The core mechanisms of civil society—freedom of speech, association, and assembly—allow peaceful and open debate on how to protect all people from harm and promote their flourishing. These human rights protections, once enacted, should shield individuals from cruelty, avoidable suffering, and interference (sometimes termed "negative freedoms" or "negative liberties"), and ensure the environment provides individuals with the minimum security, power, and resources to enable their ability to thrive (sometimes termed "entitlements" or "positive liberties"). Historian Michael Ignatieff observes that human rights protections empower the victims of past abuses by validating their right to exist free from harm (Ignatieff, 2001). Human rights, he argues, confer dignity on and give agency to those whose rights have been violated or threatened because human rights signify that they, too, are equal in their claim to the minimum conditions that support human well-being.

Scholarship on human rights originating in the Global North often emphasizes the rights of individuals, disconnected from their embeddedness in relationships to the family and community systems to which they owe basic social obligations.[6] African conceptions of human rights, by contrast, are relational in their framing; they are rooted in notions of belonging to a communal whole and on entitlements to social inclusion and connection (Kenyon, 2019, p. 167). Variants of the African philosophy of Ubuntu embody this perspective. Ubuntu philosophy suggests that our full humanity and our sustenance as social and spiritual creatures can only be realized through interdependence. Like Ubuntu philosophy, African discourse on human rights emphasizes the ties that bind African societies together in cooperative and interconnected communities to which every person rightfully belongs, and in which each has a responsibility to ensure others' belonging. Fulfilling duties to family and community are among the principal mechanisms for ensuring social inclusion. Safeguarding societal cohesion supersedes amplifying individual rights.[7] Community psychologists

Isaac and Ora Prilleltensky, in their writing on the psychological sense of mattering, describe a similar notion that they term the culture of "we-ness." They argue that our ability to thrive as individuals and achieve social equality are each difficult to attain absent such a culture: "We all have the right and responsibility to feel valued and add value, to our self and others, so that we may all experience wellness and fairness" (Prilleltensky & Prilleltensky, 2021, p. 16).

Balancing the tensions between individual and communal conceptions of human rights is not easy. Our aspirations align with those articulated in the Yogyakarta Principles (2006), an international set of human rights principles developed to ensure protection of sexual and gender minority people worldwide. We believe just societies grant individuals the means for social inclusion and belonging; provide them the material foundation for human well-being; protect them from avoidable cruelty, abuse, and suffering; and ensure their ability to contribute to civil society. Securing these rights and entitlements does not preclude the formation of cohesive societies that maximize every citizen's potential for wellness and the benefits that can be derived from unqualified community membership. In present-day reality, however, few if any societies succeed in achieving civility toward everyone.

Stigma, Discrimination, and State Repression

Stigma, discrimination, and repression of civil society often feed one another. Efforts to limit the functioning of civil society through formal and de facto means enable the neglect and undermining of people's rights and entitlements and legitimize their stigmatization and exclusion. It is largely through citizens and civil society institutions that ongoing pressure for rights and entitlements are exerted on states, and that violations of rights and entitlements are documented, held up to public scrutiny, and accountability for their redress pursued. The quality of the relationship between the state and its civil society institutions affects the quality of response to concerns of everyday life, including the HIV response (Smith, 2019). For many sexual and gender minority-led citizens and organizations in regions such as Africa and the Caribbean, that relationship is damaged, which is among the reasons bills such as the "Promotion of Proper Human Sexual Rights and Ghanian Family Values Bill" are so alarming. Rather than repair an already tenuous relationship between disenfranchised citizens and their government, bills such as this one seek to rend that tie completely.

Civil society is composed of diverse actors, from loosely organized citizen collectives and social movements to trade and professional associations to community-led and nongovernment organizations. Nurturing this rich diversity and its respectful engagement is the foundation of a civil society that thrives in its efforts to promote a better life for all citizens. Global development scholars Nicola Banks, David Hulme, and Michael Edwards use the metaphor of a natural ecosystem to characterize civil society:

> Like a natural ecosystem, civil society gains strength and sustenance from two things: one is diversity so that all angles of a problem can be tackled from service delivery to street protest; and the other is connections, so that the whole can be more than the sum of its parts and synergies can be developed from different elements. (Banks et al., 2015, p. 714)

Beginning in the mid- to late 1990s, the number of civil society institutions classified as nongovernment and community-led organizations rose sharply, driven in no small part by increases in development assistance to regions such as Africa. Development donors frequently mandate nongovernment and community-led institutions' involvement in development programs, encouraging dramatic growth in their numbers. A massive influx of AIDS-related funding to hard-hit low- and middle-income countries contributed substantially to the expansion of these types of organizations in the Global South (Morfit, 2011). Organizations rapidly shifted their attention to HIV not simply because of its enormous impact on their societies; they followed the availability of otherwise scarce resources. Indeed, some scholars point out that the influx of HIV funding was so great that it shifted needed attention away from pressing social issues and simultaneously dwarfed investment in other serious health concerns.

Explosive growth in the number of nongovernment and community-led organizations has been met by attempts by states to control and limit the influence of these organizations and, in so doing, to manage the influence of the foreigners who invest in and support them (Brass et al., 2018; Burger & Seabe, 2014; Glasius et al., 2020; Pousadela & Perera, 2021). Restrictions on nongovernment and community-led organizations—creating barriers to their registration as legal entities, placing limits on and erecting barriers to receipt of foreign funding, prohibiting engagement in certain activities—are among the strategies that governments commonly deploy to impede the functioning of these organizations and to blunt the influence of their foreign investors. For example, in August 2021, following a contentious election season, Uganda suspended the legal status of 54 nongovernment and community-led organizations, including high-profile national civil liberties watchdogs and electoral critics (Aljazeera, 2021; Biryabarema, 2021). Uganda later suspended the legal status of its leading sexual and gender community-led organizations and other allied organizations the government claimed promoted sexual and gender minority concerns.[8] In May 2019, Zimbabwe arrested seven human rights workers on charges of sedition upon their return from a human rights meeting in the Maldives (Human Rights Watch, 2019b). These human rights defenders each worked on different causes, including girls' and prisoners' rights. In Cameroon, CAMFAIDS staff were arrested in December 2021, while attempting to intervene on the behalf of an indigent transgender client who had been detained by police. Examples such as these are far too easy to find.

States in many parts of the world possess long histories of restricting and repressing sexual and gender minority groups, as we illustrate in the Introduction to this book.

In 2019, in addition to laws criminalizing same-sex sexual relationships (Chapter 1), 42 United Nations member states possessed laws limiting sexual and gender minority freedom of expression and 51 imposed legal barriers to forming and operating organizations that address sexual and gender minority concerns (International Lesbian, Gay, Bisexual, Trans, and Intersex Association, 2021). African countries accounted for 47.6% and 52.9%, respectively, of these countries, with countries in Southeast Asia and East Asia and the Pacific constituting the next largest share of nations enacting these types of restrictions. Epidemics such as HIV exacerbate these and other forms of stigma and discrimination.[9] Gender and sexual minority community-led organizations become easy scapegoats for governments attempting to draw attention away from failed or repressive policies affecting other segments of the populous (Currier, 2019).

Another common tactic to block civil society participation occurs through exclusion from high-level consultations and the fomenting of traditional and faith-based leaders to oppose calls for structural change (Smith, 2019). HIV activists increasingly express concern over shuttering civil society space, driven by appeals to nationalism and religious conservatism. Mbuso, a human rights activist who was vital to the advocacy work we later describe, explained in an interview in February 2019, that he is prohibited from speaking with government officials in the open because his organization publicly advocates for sexual and gender minority rights in Zimbabwe, a country that criminalizes sex between males:

> If now I want to go to government and say, "I'm from SRC," they won't allow me. So, even if you want to engage in other advocacy, maybe in Parliament, we need to go through maybe under National AIDS Council or MUTASA [a youth-focused NGO] or these other NGOs. They are sponsored by government.... Maybe we can go underneath and then come and say, "I'm from SRC," but straight, we can't.... Even now if I call them and say I'm SRC they say, "Ahhhhhh. That NGO for gays."

He went on to note that some government officials might be willing to have an unofficial private conversation with him, but that was the best he might hope for. Although Zimbabwe is not among African countries restricting freedom of expression or creating legal obstacles to the formation of sexual and gender minority-focused organizations, its history of silencing and sidelining such groups is well documented. In 1995, for example, the Zimbabwean government pressured the organizers of Zimbabwe's international book fair to prohibit the community-led organization, Gay and Lesbians of Zimbabwe, known as GALZ, from operating an exhibit booth. The theme of the fair that year was human rights and justice. The late president of Zimbabwe, Robert Mugabe, opened the fair that year by exclaiming:

> I find it extremely outrageous and repugnant to my human conscience that such immoral and repulsive organizations, like those of homosexuals that offend

against the laws of nature and the morals of religious beliefs espoused by society should have any advocates in our midst. (Meldrum, October 13, 2009)

Although formal legal impediments to the operation of sexual and gender minority community-led organizations may not exist in countries within the Caribbean Commonwealth, elected officials desire to maintain political distance from these groups to preserve their electability and avoid condemnation by powerful conservative religious and civic leaders. This distancing creates de facto barriers to civil society participation of sexual and gender minority organizations. Tarone, a Jamaican activist, described to me how homophobia limits sexual and gender minority people's political and civic participation. He observed that a synergistic relationship exists between the reluctance of people to make themselves vulnerable to the violence and intimidation that might result from their engaging in public forms of advocacy, on the one hand, and on the other, the extreme political wariness of Jamaican Parliamentarians to associate themselves publicly with sexual and gender minority people and their concerns:

But a gay man averagely would not be able to go like other activist groups, like the religious groups, to go before the Parliament or the Office of the Prime Minister without permit, and with placards, and telling the Prime Minister to do better. That sort of civic participation, I would say, does not take place.

    Robin: And there isn't, for example, an openly gay politician you can point to?

    This is my secret information. There is not a politician that openly lives as LBGT. There are those who are perceived. And in an instance where one was perceived to be and it came up in Parliament, underhanded comments were made in a context that would indicate his LGBT identity with words like 'fish' and 'whale.' From what I know and what I have perceived, he would have been removed from political participation because of the complication that provided or created for the party. But also, no party here wants to be aggressive on LGBT issues because they think that it may be at the expense of political victory.

Restrictions, intimidation, and exclusion push community-led organizations to adapt their public role to accommodate their national and cultural context. In exchange for safety, security, and stability, community-led organizations may find it necessary to diminish their political profile (Currier, 2012) and quiet their public relationships to other grassroots actors and social movements (Banks et al., 2015). The national political environment may force community-led organizations to operate their human rights advocacy under cover rather than in the open (Mulé, 2021), as the Ghana bill would certainly guarantee, or via organizations that are willing to act in an allied role but which are not publicly known as sexual and gender minority focused. Mulé argues that this type of repression drives community-led organizations to engage in subversive advocacy activity under the guise of HIV-related service provision.

The Foreign Aid Paradox

Scholars identify a second synergistic yet paradoxical force driving the depoliticization of nongovernment and community-led organizations, one that hampers their ability to pursue human rights advocacy and curtails their pursuit of innovative social problem solving: development aid. Banks and her colleagues (2015) assert that development aid withers nongovernment and community-led organizations' community roots and, with those roots, activism. To take on foreign aid successfully, nongovernment and community-led organizations must undergo sufficient degrees of professionalization to reassure donors that they can successfully manage funds and attain observable results. Donor preferences for certain organizational structures and forms may prompt once small community-led, membership-based, and volunteer advocacy organizations to become large, professionally staffed organizations with managerial and service delivery capacity. Donors who prefer to fund these professionalized organizations may unwittingly undermine community-led grassroots activism and community self-determination.

Professionalization and evolving to enhance service delivery capability can change community-led organizations in profound ways. Social class distance between an enlarging professional staff and constituents may emerge or increase, as those with advanced degrees become the preferred and best-paid employees. Staff who come from constituent communities or possess close ties to those communities may decrease in number, status, and influence. This may be especially pronounced in settings where sexual and gender minority people face substantial obstacles to acquiring the advanced education and professional development opportunities required to fill certain positions. Ironically, the very strengths that may have initially attracted a donor—rich community ties, intersectional inclusion, and authentic connections—may be compromised to meet donors' expectations of what features a capable organizational entity possesses. Bureaucratization and professionalization may succeed in reducing community ownership and control over the institutions that communities founded and originally led (Moreau & Currier, 2021). Communities may no longer drive the agenda, as expert-driven leadership gradually replaces membership-based governance.

Restrictive donor practices, donor dependence, and donor demands can combine to shift accountability upward from grassroots constituents to the donor community itself. The power of donors to set the agendas and terms for their fulfillment can simultaneously erode public faith in nongovernment and community-led organizations and fuel deep disillusionment among their staff (Burger & Seabe, 2014). The depoliticizing impact of donor influence is thought to be especially strong in Africa, where dependence on external foreign resources to address social problems is great (Daniel & Neubert, 2019). Concurrently, donors' preference for investing in activities that produce short-term, readily observed, and externally predetermined results further curtails community efforts to address structural inequities and transform existing social arrangements. Donor dependence may starve the evolution of innovative solutions that are grounded in and appropriate to the local context by favoring programs that reflect strategies perceived as cost-efficient and scalable (Farmer, 2005; Watkins & Swidler, 2012). Donors may require narrowly focused programs adherent to prescribed and inflexible plans. Akoni, another human rights activist from Jamaica, put it this way:

> I think engaging the community in non-HIV-related interventions impacts positively on the HIV interventions but that is not done as often because HIV donors are particularly rigid in how you spend on HIV and the kind of interventions that you have to do. And it's oftentimes very difficult to see how just providing a social space for people to engage and have fun without pricking their fingers [for an HIV test] is an HIV intervention. I think those are opportunities. But I think I have far more negative to say about what's happening than there are positive, because I think that the interventions are particularly limited.

Akoni's observations were widely shared by his colleagues from the other countries in our transnational partnership.

Programs designed from outside the community may not encapsulate what matters to people locally. Evolving to meet donor needs (or, similarly, serving as a vehicle for service delivery on the governments' behalf) may undermine the ability to operate as a progressive and constituent-based organization whose foremost function is to reimagine the local status quo and take risks (Lipsky & Smith, 1989). Human rights scholar Chidi Anselm Odinkalu (1999) cautions that the language and ideals of human rights will not resonate with African people under these circumstances. Banks and her colleagues, in contemplating the extent to which external donors may unintentionally prevent communities from determining what constitutes a locally meaningful effort, warn that "civil society may be best nurtured when donors do less: stepping back to allow citizen groups themselves dictate the agenda and to evolve structures that suit their concerns and context" (Banks et al., 2015, p. 709).

Community-led organizations that focus on securing sexual and gender minority human rights often find themselves caught in the crosshairs of state repression and the imperatives of foreign donors, without whom they would otherwise have little access to resources (Drucker, 2021). As observed by Weerawardhana,

> Very often, development aid granted to LGBTQIA rights organizations is their only form of subsistence, as their existence as citizens and their work are categorically ignored by many governments in the global South. . . . Donor-funded LGBTQIA work leads to lasting dependences, in which LGBTQIA activists often find themselves with next to no alternative than that of expanding their funding mechanisms, satisfying the exigencies of their funders and orienting their projects and initiatives in line with the priorities of their funder. This NGO-industrial complex results in an LGBTQIA rights advocacy sector which finds it difficult to connect with local contexts, or to ground their activism locally. (2021, p. 123)

Donor preferences and restrictions may undercut rather than bolster the long-term stability of the sexual and gender minority human rights activist sector and, like governments, drive organizations to engage in advocacy activities under the cover of public health initiatives and services.

Global North–Global South Relationships

Despite a strong commitment to sexual and gender minority human rights on the part of many donors, donors from the Global North can complicate the ability of African and Caribbean sexual and gender minority community-led organizations to pursue the human rights agendas of their choosing. Scholars identify several sector-specific factors that contribute to this contradiction. A major obstacle to the realization of local sexual and gender minority advocacy agendas results from the tendency of donors from the Global North to impose Eurocentric conceptions of sexuality and gender and Eurocentric language on Global South communities. Eurocentric understandings often align poorly with local cultural norms and conceptions surrounding sexuality and gender and may also be out of step with individuals' and communities' aspirations and priorities (Corey-Boulet, 2018; Currier & Cruz, 2014; Lorway, 2015). These conceptions may "unwittingly insinuate more judgements about people's sexuality that then occlude efforts to develop effective education initiatives of health policy" (Epprecht, 2009, p. 1272). Drucker observes that sexual and gender minority people in contexts like Africa and the Caribbean may be uninterested in or unable to form alternative communities separate from their families of origin because of long-standing cultural preferences about how to organize social and economic life and, in some cases, due to the material necessity of and joy found in ongoing family and community engagement. If donors adopt a narrow view of how to improve individual lives by focusing solely on sexuality and selfhood, donors risk ignoring the local community's most pressing concerns of daily living and their quest for a form of community inclusion that reflects their traditions and values. Donors may draw unwanted attention to sexual and gender minority communities through the intervention strategies they promote, exacerbating rather than mitigating the local politicization of homophobia. Conversely, they may discourage activism outright as a potential interference with obtaining short-term social service outcomes (Eveslsage, 2016; Lorway, 2015).

Health as a Point of Leverage

The effects of foreign donor dependence and government restrictions on civil society feature prominently in the operations of the public health sector in the Global South (Smith, 2019). Despite well-placed concerns about the limits of addressing sexual and gender minority human rights considerations through the vehicle of public health, in repressive political environments public health often provides a viable point of leverage to address human rights considerations that cannot otherwise be easily tackled directly (Farmer, 2005). Because governments tolerate registering sexual and gender minority community-led organizations as HIV health care providers, while simultaneously disavowing any relationship to these groups, the formation of strategic alliances through engagement with public health can sow the seeds of an enabling and equitable environment. Advancing public health provides a less confrontational means to call attention to sexual and gender minority human rights abuses and their impact on health, broadly understood, as opposed to raising these issues in ways that exacerbate their politicization. Unsurprisingly, HIV activists view their public health work as intricately tied to the defense of human rights. In some fundamental sense, HIV service provision for sexual and gender minority populations, by its very existence in repressive policy environments, is an act of defiance and form of advocacy. Providing HIV services on the frontstage can also permit innovative ways to organize action backstage.

Mental and physical health and health care are often leading concerns for sexual and gender minority communities due to discrimination, stigma, prejudice (Chapter 1), and lack of care that is affirming of their needs and concerns (Drucker, 2021). Disparities in disease burden across health issues—including depression, anxiety, suicide, drug addiction, eating disorders, and hypertension—compel advocates to health care as a locus of their work and as a point of entry for advocacy. Sexual and gender minority activists and governments understand the body, both personal and collective, as the center and source of power. For the state, attacking the body via violent action can be an effective means of social control. For activists, protecting the body is a life-or-death proposition.

Late anthropologist, physician, and human rights advocate Paul Farmer termed equity-oriented forms of public health service delivery acts of pragmatic solidarity. Pragmatic solidarity, he argued, marries the moral obligation to make common cause with people who suffer from social injustices with concrete actions to diminish the health consequences of repeated assaults to their human dignity (Farmer, 2005, p. 146). We suggest public health also provides a point of entry or leverage for raising the question of how such abuses may be prevented through transformative structural change. Farmer cautioned the key to realizing a meaningful pragmatic solidarity that advances the cause of social justice requires working through the grassroots actors and activists who are closest to the challenges of everyday life. Farmer was skeptical of the enmeshment in power of the conventional transnational charities and professionalized human rights institutions, arguing for strategies pursued in partnership with local communities, a call well familiar to community psychology.[10] Prilleltensky and Prillentensky are among the scholars who share Farmer's concern. They observe the ameliorative interventions that are typically offered via social service programs preserve the status quo because they make no attempt to upend root causes of injustice. They assert that society's elite and powerful actors possess high stakes in ameliorative approaches, noting "advocates of amelioration are always seen in a favorable light, whereas champions of transformation are regarded as troublemakers" (Prilleltensky & Prillentensky, 2021, p. 265).

Banks and her colleagues (2015) offer an alternative to Farmer's position. They propose a potential intermediary role for the professionalized nongovernment organization in pushing for upstream changes to enable the advancement of bottom-up human rights agendas. They suggest that the nongovernment organizations that have evolved away from their community foundations should act as boundary spanners or bridges among development donors, other powerful transnational nongovernment organizations, and the local community-led organizations and movements that operate in the trenches. The value of nongovernment organizations, they argue, is in their ability to act as advocates on behalf of the smaller membership-based and community-led activist organizations that are more deeply embedded in and knowledgeable of local matters. Smith provides empirical evidence that small community-led organizations can succeed in influencing national health policy in low- and middle-income country environments when powerful actors, such as the well-funded professional nongovernment organization, intervene to ensure their access to resources and seats at the table (Smith, 2019). Although this falls far short of communities setting the agenda, as Farmer envisioned, Smith's data suggest it is one way in which nongovernment organizations might increase their local relevance and community-led actors' access to those in power.

To Smith's point, the largest global providers of funds to combat the HIV epidemic in Africa and the Caribbean remain the Global Fund and PEPFAR. Each of these two international funding bodies wields considerable power in determining which nongovernment organizations receive international support and what they are expected to do as funding recipients. These two actors, along with other large Global North government and private funders, are well positioned to ensure the engagement of community-led groups in national health policy. They can require robust civil society engagement in shaping national AIDS policies through their mandated in-country intermediary structures. The Global Fund, to its credit, identifies promotion and protection of human rights as one of its strategic objectives. It has intervened to support human rights causes, such as providing emergency funding to cover the legal fees to free jailed HIV-service providers. PEPFAR requires civil society input into country-level plans and operations. In practice, however, both could do more to ensure the engagement of activists and to support their influence on national policies and practices. Critics assert that the extent of their support to civil society actors is far too limited (Hagopian et al., 2017), especially given their funding dominance in regions such as Africa and of programs targeted to sexual and gender minority people. These and other foreign donors have done too little to ensure that their funds are used in ways that protect and advance the rights of sexual and gender minority people. A recent scandal regarding the use of foreign funds speaks to these failures. In June 2021, watchdog groups uncovered that HIV providers in Kenya, Tanzania, and

Uganda provided or made referrals to "conversion" therapy (McCool, 2021), which as we noted earlier, is a widely discredited and nontherapeutic practice. Facilities offering or making referrals included those supported by USAID, UKAID, and the Global Fund.

The scale of the threat of HIV to nations in Africa and the Caribbean creates an opportunity to connect a significant public health priority with human rights considerations for sexual and gender minority people (Kenyon, 2019). HIV presents the opportunity to reveal and disrupt governments' abdication of their responsibilities to protect sexual and gender minority people from harm and provide them basic entitlements. As we have already shown (Chapter 1), inadequate consideration of the unique challenges resulting from stigma and discrimination hampers the HIV response throughout Africa and the Caribbean. Criminalization laws and a generally unfavorable social and political environment position nascent sexual and gender minority community-led organizations as essential providers of services in lieu of government and private entities, filling what might otherwise be an empty field. Sexual and gender minority community-led organizations are especially important venues for those who lack the economic means to pursue private services, among those who are willing to pursue services at all. They are also a site for connectedness and support in the face of extraordinary hostility and stigma.

Given this context, transnational alliances among local community-led organizations, local intermediaries, and transnational sexual and gender minority activists provide a promising model to pursue structural changes to enable the right to access HIV care freed from stigma, discrimination, and violence. Research suggests that transnational alliances benefit local civil society actors' ability to gain the traction needed to achieve local influence (Smith, 2019). However, the road to success in such partnerships contains many hazards. Transnational alliances, no matter how sound, may align local advocates with Western cultural imperialism and, in the case of African countries, its harrowing legacies of colonization and exploitation. For Caribbean nations, the specter of the transatlantic slave trade provides a critical backdrop to transnational alliances (Lovell, 2015). In Africa, Daniel and Neubert note that civil society includes traditional precolonial tribal and chiefly structures, as well as a significant number of faith-based organizations, all operating in parallel to postcolonial civil society structures. Traditional and religious leadership may be imbued with equal authority and legitimacy as national, regional, and local governments and civil society organizations. Within this diversity, governance structures that tilt toward authoritarianism coexist alongside structures that tilt toward democratic deliberation. Activists are enmeshed in their tribal, village, and religious communities, just as they are in postcolonial civil society organizations and social movements. To the extent that sexual and gender minority rights agendas and the alliances that support them are entangled with colonization and postcolonial models of civic organization, activists may stand accused of possessing a tenuous commitment to their local culture and communities. Transnational alliances run the risk of further breeding accusations of cultural rejection and antinationalism.

Conclusion

Navigating the complexities and tensions we have outlined in this chapter illustrates why transnational allies must be careful to avoid operating in an ahistorical vacuum and be willing to turn partnerships on their head (Corey-Boulet, 2018; Gosine, 2021). That is, they must defer to local knowledge and expertise. As Ignatieff asserts, "The only really effective rights regimes are 'local' ones, anchored in the traditions, institutions, and historical memory of national communities" (Ignatieff, 2001, p. 162). Rather than outsiders establishing the specifics of the work, transnational allies must permit the agenda to be built from the bottom up. And, in the words of Kenworthy and colleagues (2018), "studying up" these efforts is imperative.

In the remainder of this book, we describe the establishment and implementation of just this type of transnational partnership, one in which we turned the partnership on its head and put local activists in the lead. We set out with the broad objective of upending the stigma, discrimination, and violence that impede access to HIV care among gay, bisexual, other men who have sex with men, and transgender women. A human rights framework and core set of principles about how to work together guided us,[11] rather than a rigidly defined and inflexible set of prescriptions for how to enable structural change and what precisely to do to get there. Among our cardinal principles was that our partners, not us, are the experts on what is needed locally and know best how to go about achieving it. Our partnership included Ghanaian advocates whose ability to continue the work we will describe in these pages was exceedingly difficult at the time and is now under full-throttle attack. The work was no easier for our other partners, all of whom confront significant daily obstacles and operate in environments that are hostile to their efforts. In addition to Ghana, our partnership included activists from community-led organizations based in Burundi, Cameroon, Côte d'Ivoire, Jamaica, República Dominicana, and Zimbabwe. The partnership was supported by a community-led organization of activists based in the United States working under George's direction. The book centers on the work of all eight of these community-led organizations, exploring what they do and why it matters. Most of the events we describe took place between June 2016 and August 2020.

We simultaneously engaged in a systematic and collaborative effort to document the work, led by Robin. Robin set out to discover precisely what the work of these activists entails, what obstacles and challenges they face, how these obstacles are overcome, and what they can accomplish when they are permitted to follow their vision and instincts. Within the context of the HIV epidemic, neither bottom-up structural change efforts nor transnational partnerships are well-examined, with rare exception. Substantial research gaps exist on attempts to remove obstacles to HIV-related resources and promote access to sensitive and affirming HIV care for gay, bisexual, other men who have sex with men, and transgender women. Over the 12-year period spanning 2003 and 2015, just 23 investigations of structural interventions to increase accessibility, availability, or acceptability of HIV-related resources by targeting human rights–related barriers were published, only one of which addressed gay and bisexual men's access (Stangl et al., 2019). Among studies conducted in Africa, most were set in the highest-functioning democracies on the continent. We know far too little about how structural change strategies work in low- and middle-income country environments and across the wide range of political architectures, legal systems, and cultural norms reflected in these settings. This book spotlights how we went about documenting the work of the partners (see "About the Evaluation"), as we believe the approach we took, while appreciated among many quarters of the evaluation community, is often underappreciated by or unfamiliar to those outside of it. Our exploration of evaluation practice is not focused on its technical aspects, as much as it is on showing how engaged and decolonizing evaluation approaches unfold and help support human rights advocacy. Although the story we tell here is the story of the partners and relies on their voices, as witnessed by and mediated through Robin, it is also the tale of what transformative evaluation can look like on the ground.

The first time Robin met Tarone, a Jamaican activist, she asked him to characterize the political dynamics of his country on the human rights of Jamaica's sexual and gender minority citizens. He spoke at length about his perception that, in Jamaica, sexual and gender minority people were unproblematic, providing they remained socially, politically, and otherwise invisible. When it came to matters of living, Tarone indicated, that is when human rights became "tricky." Marriage. Housing. Employment. Education. Health care. Public assembly. His list of what constitutes tricky was long. It covered every aspect of the basic provisions and social protections a modern society might afford its citizens—a gay agenda, as he and his colleagues referred to it, playing on the language of Christian opponents to sexual and gender minority human rights. The way forward, Tarone argued, was a middle space carefully negotiated among local communities of activists, Jamaica's duty bearers, and the international actors who apply pressure and lend support to his community. "Politics," he concluded, "gives hope and sometimes it is not palpable or even substantive, but the idea of hope is that something that we as LGBT people latch on to."

PART II

THE MAKINGS OF PROJECT ACT

Expertise is local. MPact is only a catalyst.
—**Mohan, MPact Country Lead**

Part II describes the genesis of Project ACT. In Chapter 3, we present the origins for the conceptualization of a coordinated transnational advocacy effort to address stigma, discrimination, and violence as barriers to HIV care for gay and bisexual men and transgender women and the arduous process by which the effort secured funding. We introduce the primary community-led organizations that participated in the project and the project's leadership, describing the process by which they collaboratively selected advocacy targets and tactics. We detail how the evolving conceptualization of the project balanced local leadership against transnational coordination. In Chapter 4, we characterize the process of integrating an evaluation specialist into the transnational activist leadership team and how the partners established themselves as a learning community.

3

The Small and Mighty

Baked Into Its DNA, June 2016

I (George) was eagerly expecting the announcement. For years, MPact had lobbied the Elton John AIDS Foundation (EJAF) and the Office of the Global AIDS Coordinator (OGAC) to include gay men and transgender women in their HIV global policy and funding priorities. MPact had applied six times for EJAF funding, but without success. And then, on June 16, 2016, the announcement finally came: EJAF and OGAC jointly established a new LGBT fund that had just issued its first request for proposal (RFP). Surely, this was our chance to get a sizeable multiyear grant and to be acknowledged for the important work we were doing and wanted to continue. Activists in MPact's network had long argued that sexual and gender minorities' disproportionate disease burden could be traced to the pervasive stigma, discrimination, violence, and criminalization they endured (Chapter 1). We wanted the world to notice, and we wanted to break the silence about how the HIV pandemic was shaped by homophobic, transphobic, and other punitive laws and policies. When I received the announcement about the funding opportunity, it seemed like an advocacy win on two fronts. Two of the most influential funders in the AIDS world were at last talking openly about barriers to HIV services for gay men and transgender women. They were also putting their money where their mouths were—check and check! As MPact's executive director at the time, I saw our organization's work as perfectly aligned with this development. It felt as though all of our activism, our work, our analyses, our experiences, our thinking, our political maneuvering, our losses (and there were many), and our wins over the previous decade had led to that moment in 2016, when EJAF and OGAC issued their call for proposals. It was our time. I was sure of it.

Chapter 3 is an origin story. I (George) describe the genesis of Project ACT and the organization that birthed it. Using MPact as the example, I illustrate the struggles faced by community-led and LGBT-led organizations to secure financial support described in Chapter 2. This chapter also exposes how power operates in the context of international funding for HIV advocacy. In telling the story of how Project ACT came to be, I share my relationship to the work that Robin and I chose to undertake together with our partners. Finally, we detail how MPact selected Project ACT partners and provides an overview of partners' country contexts.

Breaking Barriers. Robin Lin Miller and George Ayala, Oxford University Press. © Oxford University Press 2024.
DOI: 10.1093/oso/9780197647684.003.0004

Making Mpact

MPact was founded in 2006 to draw global attention to the disproportionate impact HIV was having on gay and bisexual men. Everywhere in the world, the early days of AIDS were like living in a nightmare. So many of us became horribly sick. So many of us died. Some of us became activists. We founded an AIDS movement to care for our own, and to advocate for the resources that our families, employers, communities, and governments had denied to us. It was an uncertain time. It was a time of deferred dreams. When news of medical breakthroughs arrived, such as highly active antiretroviral therapy (HAART), waves of relief swept over our communities. Many of us then left our work as activists and caregivers to pick up the pieces of our lives, to return to paid work, to hit "play" on paused careers. This was certainly true for Don Baxter, an Australian AIDS activist and MPact's cofounder. But after the advent of antiretroviral medications, the Australian government began to reduce its investments in community-led HIV responses. This resulted in sharp spikes in new HIV infections among gay men. This deeply worried Don, as it worried many other gay men and their allies. Don was so troubled, in fact, that he left his job with the Australian Council for the Arts to become the executive director of the Australian Federation of AIDS Organizations. Don felt that society's response to HIV needed to be reenergized, and he came back into the movement.

Don attended the 2002 International AIDS Conference in Barcelona to meet with researchers, policymakers, funders, and other activists. There, he noticed that gay men were not publicly visible, especially in leadership roles. There were no plenaries focused on gay men, nor any openly gay speakers, despite widespread community knowledge of the heavy toll HIV was taking back home. Don knew HIV was wreaking havoc among sexual and gender minority people in Asia and Australia, and suspected strongly that it was also true in Africa, the Caribbean, Latin America, North America, and Eastern and Western Europe. Steadily, Don developed an awareness about gay men who were organizing outside of his home country and the Global North. On vacation to Southeast Asia, he connected with the Rainbow Sky Association of Thailand, an LGBT rights organization, and met Rapeepun Ohm Jommaroeng, leader of its secretariat. Don's activist mind expanded. Something had changed. In the run-up to the 2004 International AIDS Conference in Bangkok, Don flew between Australia and Thailand several times. He thought carefully with his colleagues about how lessons learned in Thailand could be shared with the international community, ultimately cementing a collaboration among the Rainbow Sky Association of Thailand, the Victorian AIDS Council, and the AIDS Council of New South Wales. Together, Don and his activist collaborators planned for a community-led satellite meeting at the 2004 conference, and it was this gay men's preconference that was my own entry into global HIV activism. About 100 people from around the world attended, and we decided there and then to create a global network centered on our communities. But it wasn't until the 2006 International AIDS Conference that the idea of a global network gained traction. Riding the high from another remarkably successful preconference event, where 300 people gathered in Toronto, the 2006 preconference organizing committee founded themselves as the steering committee of MPact (then known as the Global Forum on MSM and HIV). I was soon appointed MPact's first executive director (a story for another time).

In the intervening years before EJAF and OGAC issued the RFP in 2016, MPact built partnerships with grassroots organizations in all but four PEPFAR-funded countries. These organizations varied in size and focus, representing a cross-section of community actors working to address the HIV, health, and human rights concerns of sexual and gender minority communities. One of our principal strategies paired technical support with subcontracted funding, directly supporting country-level activists who were critical of the usual, top-down approaches to technical assistance delivered by large international nongovernment organizations. These top-down models, the activists argued, did not fully reflect the real-world conditions that grassroots activism had to navigate. International nongovernment organizations had a notorious reputation for parachuting in, training, gathering intel, and then leaving without investing further funding or deepening their community relationships. MPact's technical support philosophy, by contrast, entrusted grassroots activists via peer partnerships nurtured over time. MPact provided technical support services only after getting to know our partners and having them get to know us.

MPact's approach was baked into its DNA—as an agency founded by activists, to whose countries it was now returning with assistance. In conversation with country-level partners, we tailored technical support through cooperation with activists working on the frontlines. We familiarized ourselves with their organizations' financial, administrative, and technical capacities, as well as the policy environments they operated in. MPact's technical support services ranged from continuous needs assessment to tailored one-on-one assistance. When we couldn't connect our partners to one another for knowledge exchange and peer support—which was MPact's main technical assistance strategy and means for building a global community network of activists—we instead linked our partners to vetted, community-sensitive and acceptable, content experts.

MPact staff was diverse, with members representing four continents. To me, it was important that our partners saw their own experiences reflected on our team. In fact, compared with other major gay-led advocacy organizations situated in the Global North, MPact was rare in its racial and gender diversity. It also had a deep skills bench, an accomplishment that brought me a profound sense of pride. On my team there were former executive directors, human rights experts, physicians, artists, people with business and accounting degrees, and social media wizards. Here I was, a Puerto Rican gay man who grew up in a government subsidized housing complex in Loisaida, an economically disenfranchised New York City neighborhood, doing international work, and leading this tiny but mighty agency!

By 2015, we had expanded our technical support to reach advocacy and HIV service organizations in 31 countries. Between 2012 and 2015 alone, we managed over 90 subcontracts worth millions of US dollars. We worked with United Nations agencies to write, publish, and disseminate an important document: *Implementing*

Comprehensive HIV and STI Programs with Men Who Have Sex with Men: Practical Guidance for Collaborative Interventions (MSMIT, as it came to be called). MSMIT was the preeminent source document for HIV program planning. It was widely used in low- and middle-income countries by health ministries and program implementers to develop government grant proposals for the Global Fund to Fight AIDS, Malaria, and Tuberculosis (United Nations Population Fund et al., 2015). MPact had also expanded its support to include regional networks in Asia and the Pacific, Eastern Europe and Central Asia, Latin America and the Caribbean, the Middle East and North Africa, and sub-Saharan Africa. By 2016, MPact had instigated a global movement to address homophobic stigma and discrimination through strengthening public health policies and alleviating funding disparities. Working at the intersection between the HIV and LGBT rights sectors, we were linked to 133 community-led organizations across 73 countries

Partnership, community-led, knowledge-informed, unapologetically open and affirming of sexual and gender minority people—these characteristics were not the only things distinguishing MPact from the big international nongovernment organizations. We truly understood advocacy. For us, effective advocacy strategies that are designed to remove barriers to HIV services are characterized not by their ability to proceed along a predicted track, but by their capacity to adapt to changing circumstances. The most effective community-led organizations are not defined by a single measurable goal, but by clearly articulated organizing principles that can be adapted to hundreds of situations, including those in countries that are hostile to sexual and gender minority communities. For MPact, robust advocacy organizations working at the intersection between the HIV and LGBT rights sectors should have a record of innovating and reorganizing when their tactics don't work as well as they should, or as well as they once did. MPact's own evaluation plans for its partner organizations had moved beyond single measurable goals to detect wider patterns of influence. This philosophy, built on our decade of experience, informed the proposal we made to EJAF and OGAC in response to the LGBT Fund announcement.

The team at MPact saw the LGBT Rapid Response Fund as an opportunity to strengthen LGBT community capacity, especially as it seeks to combat structural violence motivated by homophobia and transphobia. Using a within-network, partnership model, MPact proposed a six-step process to EJAF and OGAC. The process would quickly and efficiently administer up to 80 new subgrants with community-led groups working across 29 countries. We also proposed widening the monitoring efforts of the LGBT Rapid Response Fund's progress—while the funders wanted to monitor individual subgrantees against their prenegotiated key performance indicators, we suggested evaluating the funded portfolio's aggregate returns on investments. (We proposed treating efforts to remove barriers to HIV services for sexual and gender minority people as a portfolio of distinct, properly vetted "bets," on the assumption that some strategies would be successful, while others may not be.) MPact's within-network, peer-led partnership approach would have invested in a wide range of organizations, strategies, scenarios, and issues. We strongly believed that failing to fund an unconventional, untried, homegrown strategy, and community-led organizations would be a lost opportunity in the fight against HIV—just as significant of a loss as funding a strategy inappropriate to a local context or specific situation.

Pushback, July 18–22, 2016

Our proposal was rejected. I received the news during the XXI International AIDS Conference in Durban. At first, I was stunned. Then I was sad, confused, and finally mad. I had received rejection notices scores of times before, but this time it felt different, somehow personal. These were hard emotions to contain at a conference of 15,000 people, and I worried that people might notice the physical upset I wore on my body. I could hardly lose myself in the crowd, either. For better or worse, people knew who I was: George Ayala, the executive director of that global H-O-M-O-S-E-X-U-A-L network. In retrospect, what stung most was the funders' decision to award US$4 million to the International HIV/AIDS Alliance, now known as Frontline AIDS. Founded in 1993, Frontline AIDS is a large, professional international nongovernment organization based in the resort city of Brighton in England. The organization was notorious among advocates and activists for its egregious strategy of establishing satellite hubs in low-income countries to access funding intended for local, community-led organizations. Frontline AIDS were far bigger than MPact, and not LGBT-led. At a Durban press conference, EJAF and OGAC planned to announce Frontline AIDS as the LGBT Fund inaugural's grant recipient. *Frontline AIDS*?! I felt a strong urge to scream.

Soon, I got my chance. One afternoon, in a busy hallway at the Inkosi Albert Luthuli International Convention Center, I crossed paths with the senior program officer overseeing the LGBT Fund. I asked for a few minutes of his time. We stepped to the side of the hallway to find what little privacy we could. "I'm sorry MPact wasn't selected," he said, quick to express his condolences.

I was as quick to reply. "We didn't receive a score," I said. "Is it possible to see reviewer remarks? I'd like to see feedback to better understand what we did wrong."

"I can send to you their review when I get back to the office," he said. "I want you to know that your proposal was ranked second by the reviewers."

Perhaps, he thought, I would feel better knowing MPact was runner-up. I didn't. Not willing to accept the decision, I took the only position I could. "I have to say I'm surprised and utterly disappointed that EJAF and OGAC decided to give the inaugural award to a beltway bandit and not to MPact." I said "beltway bandits" is reference to what the large, international nongovernment organizations were often called. With the conference "high" the program officer might have been feeling now long gone, I went on: "Does EJAF really want to risk losing face with their constituencies by announcing that the first award of the newly founded LGBT Fund is going to a large, professional, UK-based, technical assistance provider that isn't even LGBT-led?"

The program officer, whom I considered a friend and supporter of MPact's work, was stunned at the directness of my words. I was, too. I knew I was taking a risk in making such an unabashed intervention. But I was buoyed by MPact's reputation, history, and the knowledge that our proposal was ranked a close second. The program officer seemed shaken, but he patiently took in the feedback and promised to be in touch soon. I left this brief, but terse, encounter relieved to have expressed my upset and prepared to put the entire situation behind me.

Much to my surprise, however, the program officer called the next morning. He confessed that after our encounter he had returned to his room and wept. He was so moved by our brief conversation that he made calls as soon as he could to his counterparts at OGAC, who were somehow able to find an additional US$1.5 million in available funds. This was less than half (37.5%) the amount awarded to Frontline AIDS, but rather than managing the LGBT Rapid Response Fund—which Frontline AIDS would still go on to do—EJAF and OGAC's leadership now wanted MPact to support advocacy initiatives in sub-Saharan Africa and the Caribbean aimed at removing barriers to HIV services. "It's important to us that MPact stays true to its mission as an advocacy organization," the project officer said. He then asked me to develop an entirely new 2-year scope of work and budget. They now planned to announce two inaugural recipients of their LGBT Fund at their press event, he said, and that I should be there. I felt vindicated, and relieved that MPact would leave Durban with new funding. I was also thrilled that I could announce the award at MPact's 10-year anniversary celebration later that week in the Global Village.

A Conspicuous Silence

Luckily, I had packed a jacket and some khakis and could dress "business casual." I needed to look my best—it would be my first time meeting a celebrity. A star. Sir Elton John! On the day of the press conference, Sir Elton walked around with a gaggle of underlings and security guards. Ambassador Dr. Debra "Debbie" Birx was on stage, too—the United States Global AIDS Coordinator and Special Representative for Global Health Diplomacy. I had shared the stage with the ambassador on previous occasions. She had visited MPact's office in downtown Oakland, California, when MPact organized a meeting for her with West African activists, gay men leading the HIV response in their respective countries. We had wanted to bring West African HIV challenges to her attention, chief among them being the daily harassment and violence that sexual minority people endured to secure their basic needs and their HIV-related services. The ambassador was kind, personable, and engaged. When I saw her on stage, she greeted me warmly, as she often did. Sir Elton, however, was distant. He seemed happy to be there but less "leaned in." We did our thing and showed up for the press. Statements were made. Congratulations were extended and gratitude given in return. Sir Elton was quoted as having said:

> Establishing the LGBT Fund between EJAF and PEPFAR is something we've worked towards for a long time in our attempts to make a real and lasting difference in HIV

awareness, education, and prevention. Just earlier today we visited ANOVA clinic, a project both EJAF and PEPFAR have funded in the past. The work they are doing through their "We the Brave" programme, the first large scale campaign ever in South Africa to address both prevention and treatment issues in an affirming, non-judgmental and sex positive way, is something for us all to be incredibly proud of. We look forward to building long standing relationships with the International HIV/AIDS Alliance (The Alliance) and the Global Forum on MSM and HIV (MSMGF)[1] in a similar way. (United States Department of State, 2016)

Looking back, I realize that Sir Elton, the queerest man on the planet, did not mention gay men. Nor did he utter the words "transgender women." He did not speak about MPact's work. In fact, he drew press attention to EJAF's ongoing support of the ANOVA clinic. An extraordinary clinic indeed, but weren't we all there to celebrate the inaugural recipients of the LGBT Fund? I would like to think that Sir Elton John's conspicuous silence was like that of many people in his role. His silence at that moment felt like the silence I had often experienced in the HIV and international development spaces. That silence was frustratingly familiar and deafening. It was the silence I experienced from people who must engage with the bigger donors and the bigger dignitaries—those who keep foundations like EJAF afloat. I know that hustle. To get the big money, you must give the big donors what they want, and the big donors want to feel they are helping the innocent and downtrodden. Sexual and gender minority people don't fit into that trope—the needs of gay men and transgender women are too taboo to discuss openly and directly, lest we risk unwelcome scrutiny and stigma from the mainstream. And when this happens, funding that once flowed freely could be reduced to a trickle. Ambassador Birx, however, was a bit more direct: "We stand with and for LGBT people everywhere who are too often forced into the shadows and lack access to HIV services," she said. "Together we are putting our words into action to reach LGBT people with HIV services and stop stigma in its tracks." I don't remember giving a statement myself. Perhaps because I was lost in the fanfare and performance, or perhaps I wasn't asked to give one. Nevertheless, I left South Africa happy in the knowledge that MPact's reputation as a strong advocacy actor was being taken seriously by two of the biggest HIV funders in the world. At least Sir Elton John knew us by name, if not by reputation. Later I learned that the US$1.5 million we were to receive came not from the LGBT Fund itself, as I had assumed, but from crumbs that the ambassador and her team had found. The press conference now made sense in ways that it hadn't before. Although the US$1.5 million was a consolation prize, I was going to take it.

The Wait, November 2016

When Hillary Rodham Clinton lost the United States' presidential election to Donald Trump in the fall of 2016, getting the promised funding to MPact became a complicated dance. There was concern that Ambassador Birx's budget would be scru-tinized for savings, which was how it had been able to commit the funding in the first place: budget dust. Moreover, it became exceedingly difficult for OGAC to fund MPact directly. Until that point, MPact had never received direct funding from the United States government. MPact was not one of the large international nongovernment or-ganizations with dedicated, fully staffed, administrative and finance units, adept at processing United States government contracts. Senior staff at Birx's office were con-cerned about overwhelming MPact with due diligence requirements and a mountain of paperwork, distracting the organization from its core work. Moving funds directly to EJAF also wasn't an option. Ultimately, a convoluted solution was concocted to move funds through a familiar, mutually agreed-upon, third-party intermediary that already held contractual relationships with the United States government—UNAIDS. Funds from the United States would move to UNAIDS through a modification of an existing scope of work. But UNAIDS was also unable to directly fund MPact, for the same reasons that OGAC couldn't. Given the size of the award, MPact would have been compelled by the technocrats at UNAIDS to undergo an onerous prequalifica-tion process to receive the funds. (UNAIDS is not a funder, but rather fancies itself as a technical support entity whose mission is to lead, strengthen, and support the response to the HIV epidemic. Its funding comes from governments, and its biggest funder by far is the United States.) For a small overhead fee that would be subtracted from MPact's total award, UNAIDS agreed to move the funds to EJAF, who would then directly fund us.

As the United States presidency transitioned from one administration to another, there was growing concern that the window of opportunity to move funds from OGAC to MPact, via UNAIDS and EJAF, would quickly close. Those worries were compounded by the fact that the Trump administration would be less friendly to multilateral organizations like UNAIDS, and less friendly to LGBT causes. They were. By far.

MPact found itself chasing after the funds as they moved from institution to insti-tution, an awkward but necessary role given how lumbering large bur-eaucracies can be. MPact had to ensure that the various parties were communicating with one another in a clear and timely manner. But its efforts were in vain, and the window did close. Funding for the project would not arrive until 2018—nearly 2 years after that terse conversation with the EJAF project officer at the Durban conference. We hounded, even henpecked, OGAC, UNAIDS, and EJAF for 2 long years.

Planning While Waiting: The Project ACT Transnational Partners

The MPact team used those 2 years to pivot direction and introduce something novel to its approach. I decided to bring MPact's three programs together—programs, policy, and communications—to support our work at country level. I assigned country leads, each of whom would assess the capacity needs of the community-led organization they were paired with; manage the contract; broker other resource needs and advocacy opportunities at national, regional, and global levels when appropriate; deliver technical assistance; link their country partner to other activists; facilitate peer exchange; and advocate on organizations' behalf when called to do so. Because the MPact staff was small and insanely busy, we had to narrow the list of focus countries. We examined existing staff portfolios and asked ourselves: Which of our current partners are working to eliminate barriers to health care access? How many are there? Where do they work and with which community? If our EJAF program officer were to call, would our partners be able to start quickly? Which of our partners play well with others? We needed to think these issues through carefully.

There was a bit of back-and-forth among MPact, OGAC, and EJAF regarding our geographical focus. OGAC and EJAF each had a list of priority countries. The OGAC's priority countries were based on international market interests and policy goals. Funding through OGAC, which is housed in the United States Department of State, is considered an instrument of diplomatic relations, in service of market interests. The basis for EJAF's country priorities was less clear. In retrospect, they may have been influenced by the philanthropic ecosystem at the time, or by Sir Elton's personal wishes. The two lists overlapped and were published in EJAF's request for proposals. Fortunately, MPact had partnerships with community-led organizations and activists in all but four of the countries listed. Our next task was to figure out a sweet spot: a list of countries that satisfied each stakeholder involved.

For MPact, adhering to our partnership model was paramount. We wanted to work with organizations we knew, who had the financial capacity to receive subgrants from MPact, however small. Safety was another strong consideration, because of the type of work we envisaged. None of us wanted to work somewhere with a high possibility of violence and arrest. Nor did we wish to place our partners at even greater risk than they already faced by introducing a particularly high-risk project. We ended up selecting countries where MPact had existing relationships with the LGBT community, and where access to HIV services was seriously compromised by criminalization, stigma, discrimination, and violence. We focused on countries where there were fewer international donor investments to grassroots communities—the absence of which, from our perspective, posed a serious risk to HIV service access for gay and bisexual men and transgender women. To narrow our choices, we reviewed our entire African and Caribbean portfolio, ruling out places where our relationships were too new in their development, or where the in-country situation was too volatile to introduce a rapid-start advocacy initiative (see Figure 3.1).

The team at MPact knew right from the start that we wanted to deepen our relationships in Cameroon. It was already a priority country for our colleagues at EJAF and OGAC, given HIV's impact in the country's sexual and gender minority communities. Two of our team, Nadia and Johnny, had lobbied for years about the need to expand our work in West and North Africa. They were both French speakers, and personally familiar with these regions—Nadia having led a renowned community-led

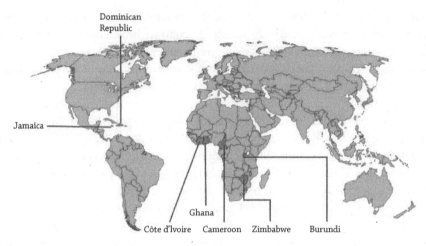

Figure 3.1 Map of Project ACT countries

organization that ran HIV programs for sexual and gender minority people in Morocco, her home country, and Johnny having founded a regional network of sexual minority people from his home country, Lebanon. Nadia had already worked with the leadership at Affirmative Action in Cameroon, having advocated with them to UNAIDS and the Global Fund for stronger assistance during PEPFAR country planning and negotiations. Affirmative Action was organizationally strong and well respected at the country and regional levels. Its mission was strongly aligned with MPact's mission. Their leadership was trusted by their constituents and had a reputation for being reliable.

In Cameroon, as is the case with large swathes of West Africa, gay men, and other men who have sex with men, experience high HIV case rates and violence. Cameroon is among the most violent countries in which a sexual or gender minority person can live, with thousands of hate crimes documented annually. During the years leading up to Project ACT, there was a rash of attacks on LGBT communities. The offices of a human rights lawyer were ransacked, resulting in the theft of confidential legal files. Assailants set fire to the offices of Alternatives Cameroun, a sister community-led organization to Affirmative Action. Numerous LGBT rights defenders and service providers received death threats, and one was murdered (Chapter 1). As a result, organizations providing services to sexual and gender minority people were forced to suspend their services (Beck et al., 2015). By the time Project ACT began, these organizations had resumed their programs, albeit in the face of continued violence and harassment. And although we wanted to avoid working in dangerous settings, the need and possible positive outcome from doing so in Cameroon outweighed the risks.

Affirmative Action, our partner of choice, is a community-led organization that launched in 2008 and was legally registered in 2010. Based in Cameroon's capital city of Yaoundé, the organization emerged from a local clinic, where several of Affirmative Action's founders volunteered as peer outreach workers. Its founder, Kenzo, mobilized four fellow outreach workers around his vision for a national membership organiza-tion that would address the health and human rights needs of gay and bisexual men. According to Guy, one of those four workers, Kenzo, wanted to "create something for our community by our community." In an interview with Robin, Kenzo dated his commitment to creating something for, and by, gay men to 1990:

> It all started in the year 1990, when we came to notice that there were more MSMs and gay men than what we thought in this country. Some MSMs started coming out and standing out as gay men; because there is a difference between being a man who has sex with men and the stigma of having sex with a man, being MSM [on the one hand] and being a gay man, someone who clearly affirms himself as a gay [on the other] . . . I thought that it would be wise for me to create an organization like Affirmative Action. And the aim of the organization was to reduce the incidence of HIV/AIDS and the number of people dying of HIV. And to improve the situation or conditions of gay men living [in] denial.

The five men began their efforts without any funding, carrying out a modest number of local activities. Gaston, another of the five, described for Robin that period as one of relentless work with "not even enough money to pay for a cab." Much of that work focused on getting gay men tested and connected to HIV care. Gaston said of those early efforts:

> We did everything possible to help our peers. I can remember my very first mis-sion. . . . I was tasked with seeking my MSM and gay men peers, to bring them to accept the need to get tested and to get treatment in order to have undetectable viral load. It was my pleasure to always convince them to come to assist with our meetings. And, at that time, we even organized some picnics. We all contributed to have picnics. So, this I can say is my greatest achievement because it is really rewarding to see some of my peers today living a very wholesome and healthy life, even [though] they have HIV. And when you look at them today, you can't even im-agine that they are HIV patients.

As the group began to attract support, funders required Affirmative Action to change its management structure. Although the organization preserved many features of a member-led institution, their primary funders, PEPFAR and the Global Fund, pushed them to adopt a hierarchical structure. Their 157 members still pay annual dues, form a general assembly to elect a president every 2 years, and contribute much of the organization's volunteer labor. But there are also paid staff—9 in the main of-fice in Yaoundé and 18 project-specific staff spread throughout nine regions of Cameroon—who interact with the funders and manage the group's projects. To carry out its work in the field, Affirmative Action collaborates with 20 small LGBT-led or-ganizations, including Avenir Jeune d'Ouest, acting as the financial intermediary and accountability agency to connect these smaller groups with international donors.

To strengthen our West African focus, we wanted to include other nations in Project ACT. First, we chose Ghana, and then, very hesitantly, Côte D'Ivoire. To strengthen our West African focus, we wanted to include other nations in Project ACT. First, we chose Ghana, and then, very hesitantly, Côte D'Ivoire. In Ghana—with its hostile climate toward LGBT people that we describe in Chapter 2—we invited a rights-focused organization based in Accra to lead our work. We do not name them here because of deteriorating safety conditions for sexual and gender minority activists and their allies (Chapter 2). Our Ghanaian partner was founded in 1998 to address human rights abuses targeted toward youth and other marginalized people, including those at high-risk of HIV infection. The organization's core methodologies are rooted in popular education strategies. Throughout its history, the organization has prioritized a focus on HIV and its impact on gay and bisexual men. Unlike several other partners, a substantial part of their effort is direct service provision, usually coordinated with mainstream service providers in Accra and surrounding areas. It has a long-standing leadership, and many of its staff are LGBT people. It is among the activist groups that routinely fight against LGBT human rights violations in Ghana, playing a significant role in combating such abuses. I asked Stephen Leonelli to serve as country lead for our work in Ghana. Stephen earned a master's degree in public policy from Harvard Kennedy School. He understood international human rights mechanisms and how important it was for organizations like our partner to focus on United Nations–level advocacy while simultaneously working at the country level. Stephen is methodical and deferential to the needs of local partners. With his strategic deliberateness, I knew he could navigate Ghana's political sensitives and safety concerns.

We were hesitant about working in Côte D'Ivoire. Prior attempts to partner with its most visible community-led organization, Alternative Côte D'Ivoire, were hampered by uneven and sometimes difficult communications, and we found them to be stand-offish. Based in Abidjan, Alternative was founded at the same time as Affirmative Action. As a visible LGBT community-led organization in the city, it has endured repeated attacks over its brief history. Côte d'Ivoire is a country wracked by widespread anti-LGBT violence. Like our other ACT partners, its staffing levels routinely grow and shrink depending on funding. When Project ACT began, it had 16 employees. With a broad mission, Alternative addresses issues of concern to lesbian and bisexual women, as well as the needs of gay, bisexual, and transgender communities. Its funding, however, is largely HIV-focused and on the needs of gay, bisexual, and other men who have sex with men. Much like Affirmative Action, its growth is attributable to funding from foreign actors. Soon after Alternative organized in 2010, PEPFAR awarded US$1.7 million to Heartland Alliance International for improving access to HIV testing and care among Abidjan's gay and bisexual men and sex worker communities. Heartland subcontracted much of that work to fledgling groups, including Alternative (Thomann, 2016), permitting Alternative to rent their first offices and purchase computers, basic office equipment, and furniture. Although they are not structured as a membership organization, Alternative remains community-led and community-staffed, under the leadership of their founder. Johnny, with support from Nadia, volunteered to serve as its country lead.

In our country portfolio review, Jamaica and República Dominicana were the only Caribbean countries in which we had long-standing partnerships. Omar had worked with organizations in both countries. A native of El Salvador, Omar had links with dozens of organizations in the Latin American and Caribbean regions. Most Caribbean governments do not collect data on violence directed at sexual minority people and, as is common everywhere in the world, many cases of violence go unreported. Community-led organizations and human rights defenders are thus often left in the unpleasant position of documenting violent incidents on their own. For example, between 2009 and 2012, one community-led organization in Jamaica documented 231 reports of anti-LGBT assaults, physical attacks, and displacement from homes (Inter-American Commission on Human Rights, 2012). In 2015, a coalition of Jamaican LGBT and human rights groups joined forces to produce a shadow report outlining human rights violations against sexual minority people. The shadow report was submitted for consideration at the 116th Session of the Human Rights Committee. Violations laid out in the report included evidence that Jamaican authorities had done too little to prevent, prosecute, and punish violent attacks and sexual assault against LGBT people, including cases where the police were either the perpetrators or did nothing to intervene.

To do the work of Project ACT in Jamaica, we turned to the first and best-known national LGBT human rights organization on the island. J-FLAG is based in the capital city of Kingston and was part of the coalition responsible for the 2015 shadow report. Founded in 1998, J-FLAG was established to advance a human rights agenda for LGBT people, one that was intentionally framed on systemic repression of LGBT people rather than the HIV epidemic (Lovell, 2016). J-FLAG's priorities are legal reform, offering support services to victims of violence and discrimination, and providing rights-focused educational outreach to the public and the LGBT community. The organization had a policy-savvy staff of 14 when Project ACT began, many of whom have advanced training in law and public policy and extensive national-level experience as legal and policy advocates. J-FLAG addresses a breadth of policy areas that affect health and well-being, from homelessness and housing policies to employment discrimination policies, to educational reforms, to the size of the national health care budget. In their conversations with Robin, Akoni characterized J-FLAG's broad focus and constant surveillance of policy advocacy opportunities as vital to their ultimate success in advancing a human rights agenda:

> What we hear on a regular basis from the community is a desire to have freedom to exist, to be, to live peacefully in their homes, in their communities, to exist peacefully at work and at school and other spaces. And, for a lot of people, that means addressing whatever impediments there might be that impact on them in that regard. And so, for some people it is sometimes the buggery law, in part because that is what LGBT advocates tend to talk about. For other people, it's about addressing

workplace discrimination, addressing all the other aspects of laws and policies that impact on them negatively in that way.

Akoni believes that health care quality and access is tied to these other aspects of life—how legislation is created, the translation of legislation into administrative policy, and how such policies are implemented on the ground. Jahmar, a J-FLAG policy analyst, put it this way when Robin interviewed him in 2018: "We're saying 'Yes. We do have a gay agenda, and this is what it is. It's very inclusive. It talks about things like housing, family, education.'"

In the República Dominicana, we sought to partner with a subsidiary of the HIV-focused service provider Amigos Siempre Amigos to lead Project ACT. Amigos Siempre Amigos was established in 2005 to advocate for LGBT rights, increase civic and political participation of LGBT people, and ensure that high-quality HIV health care is available to gay men and transgender women. Throughout its history, Amigos Siempre Amigos has been a vital source of training for grassroots activists and an effective advocate for legal reform. They are widely recognized for contributing to Gay Pride celebrations, establishing an International LGBT Film Festival, and supporting LGBT people as political candidates. Reflecting the service orientation of their parent organization, they have also invested heavily in training HIV health care providers to be more competent in serving gay men and transgender women. Although the República Dominicana lacks a criminalization law, public decency laws are used to limit daily freedoms of sexual and gender minority people and to undermine their safety. As a result, sexual and gender minority people face violence and discrimination, including hate crimes, arbitrary arrests, extortion by police, and lack of access to essential services and employment. Such hate crimes are not codified in Dominican law. Sexual orientation and gender identity are ignored in official investigations. Like many places worldwide, violence directed at members of the LGBT community is enacted with impunity.

Before our final two partners were identified, the MPact team convened virtual planning meetings with our first five partners. These early meetings reviewed EJAF's and OGAC's requests and discussed the project's overall goals, programmatic foci, and division of labor. We began to remap the program approach. All partners had one thing in common: They either ran, or wanted to run, initiatives that focused on expanding access to HIV prevention, care, and treatment services for sexual minority people. All partners, too, viewed access to health care as a human right. This early common principle was critical for holding the group of otherwise disparate advocacy actors together, and we built from there. MPact staff realized that each country partner approached their work differently, and necessarily so. Each partner adopted distinct tactics and devised advocacy strategies unique to their national contexts and local circumstances. How could we craft a scope of work that acknowledged the complexity of this portfolio yet also remained legible to our funder? Our solution was to cluster similar advocacy programs together. There were three: policy and legal barriers to HIV-related services; stigma and discrimination in health care settings; and safety and security measures to protect LGBT people from violence. These program "buckets" became interventions aimed at changing policies at the health care facility level, changing public perceptions in mainstream media coverage of sexual minority people, and leveraging international human rights instruments to create trickle-down change.

We needed to give our reimagined project a name. The team at MPact was remarkably adept at creating punchy acronyms for funders. Mohan was the mastermind behind "Project ACT." It stands for Advocacy and other Community Tactics. In our mission to break down barriers to HIV services for gay men and transgender women, our team led with advocacy, centered community, and honored activists' strategic prowess in its name choice for the initiative. Our partners loved that the name signaled action. And with that seal of approval, Project ACT was born. It was 2017. The initiative was coalescing. We were ready to go. But funds had not materialized—we were back to hounding.

We Have to Move Fast, Spring 2018

The funds finally arrived at MPact in the late spring of 2018. The team was relieved. The partners we had engaged across five countries had nearly given up hope that Project ACT would finally get launched. We assumed the funds would arrive weeks after the award announcement, but the wait turned out to be months. Nearly 2 years. We only had five partners named, and Robin was due to join us any day. We had to move quickly. The pressure to get going now felt immense, given the project's short 24-month timeframe, and the clock had started ticking the minute the funds arrived—via the ridiculously circuitous path our funders insisted upon—in our bank account. We quickly onboarded two more community-led organizations, one from Zimbabwe, as we had hoped, and one from Burundi.

Zimbabwe had always been at the top of our list, due in no small part to our long-standing and close partnership with Gays and Lesbians of Zimbabwe (GALZ). GALZ was involved in MPact's founding 10 years prior and was now leading a sensitivity training program for health care providers in southeastern Africa. On MPact's team, Mohan held this part of our broader portfolio. An Indian national from Chennai, Mohan is a trained physician. He authored MPact's first health care training curriculum, which MPact successfully piloted in Latin America and Africa. He spent countless hours in Zimbabwe to learn with, and from, activists there. Zimbabwe's hostility toward its LGBT citizens is often told through well-documented stories of enduring harassment GALZ has faced. It is one of the oldest organizations fighting on these issues in Africa, and an organization we highlighted in Chapter 2 for enduring repeated attacks and harassment by the late Zimbabwean leader, Robert Mugabe, and his government. Although GALZ would have been the obvious partner for Project ACT, their dance card was too full, and they could not take on more work. If not GALZ, then who? We had little time. If we wanted a Zimbabwean partner, we would have to identify an alternative organization. Mohan asked staff members at GALZ for their advice. Without hesitation, they recommended the Sexual Rights Centre (SRC).

SRC is headquartered in Zimbabwe's second largest city, Bulawayo, a faded industrial center on the border of the Matabeleland North and Matabeleland South provinces. Founded in 2007, the organization employs a core staff of 13. It also hosts six community-led collectives, two comprised of male and female sex workers, two of young gay and bisexual men, one comprised of transgender people, and one of lesbian and bisexual women. The collectives are deeply engaged in many of SRC's activities and develop and implement activities of their own. The collectives are SRC's mechanism for building its grassroots base, mobilizing constituents, and creating supportive space. SRC views its role as assisting the collectives to find their advocacy voice. Mbuso, who has been part of the organization from its founding, describes the early years of SRC as a search for people who could create a movement to fight stigma. (Historically, patient health advocacy has been a mainstay activity.)

At the start of Project ACT, SRC found itself at a major transition point. Its founding executive director and all his managerial staff had abruptly quit, departing with every record and even the computers. Penya, a seasoned leader, with strong connections to national and regional policy apparatus, took the helm at the beginning of 2018. Recounting those first weeks, she had no easy way to ascertain what the organization was beholden to do. She had nothing to go on but what remaining staff, like Mbuso, and long-term volunteers could help her piece together. Penya set about recreating the organization's most basic systems, shifting its culture toward team-oriented collaboration, and deepening the collectives' engagement in all aspects of the organization's functioning. According to staff and collective members, Penya is something of a miracle worker, rebuilding SRC in a transformational style that cemented their own loyalty to the organization and secured the loyalty of the wider community. The timing of Project ACT was fortuitous, according to Penya, as it could contribute to her ongoing efforts to reestablish SRC as a well-functioning national advocate for sexual and human rights. The project, she said, could help SRC become more responsive to those constituents who have stressed the need to address structural stigma and discrimination, and, for the first time in its recent history, would allow SRC to attempt this in a meaningful way.

MPact had never worked in Burundi, and MPact's staff and I were wary. In 2009, the Burundian government passed legislation criminalizing same-sex sexual relations, an act punishable by imprisonment (Human Rights Watch, 2009). Shortly after the law was enacted, the government engaged in a vicious campaign against the LGBT community. High-ranking officials included homophobic rants in public speeches, describing homosexuality as a curse. In keeping with a familiar pattern, acts of violence increased, including assaults carried out by police. At the time, there were delicate bilateral discussions taking place between the governments of Burundi and the United States about PEPFAR funding. OGAC and one of their grantees, a large international nongovernment organization, lobbied hard to have us include Burundi.

They knew LGBT organizing was nascent in Burundi and wanted MPact to provide support. I was heartened to know that one of the so-called beltway bandits had assessed the situation in Burundi with sensitivity. And I took pride from the fact that the beltway bandit wanted our help. They also wanted Burundian community voices that could represent sexual minority people and discuss their HIV needs.

The partner organization from Burundi that we engaged is headquartered in Bujumbura. For their safety, given the circumstances in their home country, we will say no more about them here.[2] This is a difficult choice because their contributions to Project ACT are many. Yet conditions in Burundi for HIV-focused work steeply deteriorated as Project ACT commenced, a trend which continues. Throughout Project ACT, our partners in Burundi operated under intense police scrutiny. The staff were surveilled as they went about their daily work, organizing other community-led groups. They could not gather in groups of more than five without running afoul of the police, relying instead on a cell-like structure and limited online activity. At one point, Pierre, who spearheaded critical aspects of the work, seriously considered seeking temporary asylum in a nearby country for his safety. I asked Stephen to lead our Project ACT work in Burundi. Given his knowledge of human rights mechanisms at the United Nations, he was an obvious choice.

By focusing on these seven countries, we succeeded in choosing collaborating partners based in low-income countries with poorly managed HIV epidemics among gay and bisexual men and transgender women. The HIV epidemics in five of these seven countries ranked among the worst in the world when our collaboration began (see Table 3.1). As we alluded to earlier, each country also exhibited extremely hostile social and political climates for the human rights of sexual minorities and gender nonconforming people. Four of the African countries rank in the bottom quartile of the 174 countries on the William's Institute's scale of societal acceptance of sexual and gender minorities; all five African countries are below the median on this measure (Flores, 2019). Five of our countries have laws criminalizing same-sex sexual relations, and the remaining two criminalize public displays of same-sex sexuality. We had our work cut out for us.

I was nervous about Robin's first visit. Although she and I remained friends for 4 decades, we hadn't worked together outside of forming alliances at research meetings. I admired Robin immensely and respected her views and her assessments. I still do. Now she was coming to MPact, an organization that I deeply cared for. But our staff had minimal and uneven evaluation experience. Many conflated case studies with evaluation. Donor-imposed evaluation requirements are often designed to determine compliance with contractual obligations, and nothing more. These are often exercises in appeasing the funder, unrelated to the team's interests or learning needs. Knowing this, some staff nevertheless simply submitted to donor subjugation. I often wonder whether their submission was simply fatigue, given their enormous work responsibilities, or whether they slipped into that state of learned helplessness common among community-led organizations hungry for funding. I was worried about what Robin would think.

Table 3.1 Characteristics of Project ACT Partner Countries at the Start of the Project in 2018

	Burundi	Cameroon	Côte d'Ivoire	República Dominicana	Ghana	Jamaica	Zimbabwe
Former colony of	Germany (1891–1916) Belgium (1916–1962)	Germany (1864–1919) France (1919–1960) England (1919–1961)	France (1843–1960)	Spain (1492–1725) United States (1916–1924)	Portugal (1471–1642) Netherlands (1598–1872) Sweden (1650–1663) Denmark, Norway (1663–1850) Germany (1682–1720) England (1867–1957)	Spain (1493–1655) England (1655–1962)	England (1893–1980)
Population size (in millions)	11.9	26.5	26.4	10.8	31	2.9	14.9
Life expectancy (in years)	61	59	57	74	64	74	61
Total AIDS cases	82,000	540,000	460,000	70,000	330,000	40,000	1,300,000
Adult HIV (15–49) prevalence	1.0%	3.6%	2.6%	.9%	1.7%	1.9%	12.7%
Estimated HIV prevalence—gay/bisexual men	4.8%	20.7%	12.3%	4.0%	18.0%	29.8%	31.0%

Estimated HIV prevalence—transgender women	Unknown	Unknown	Unknown	Unknown	Unknown	Unknown	Unknown
Criminalization law(s)	Yes	Yes	No	No	Yes	Yes	Yes
Social acceptance of LGBTQI people Country rank ($n = 174$)	160	145	127	55	141	93	149
Democracy Index[a]	2.33 Authoritarian	3.28 Authoritarian	4.15 Hybrid regime	6.54 Flawed democracy	6.63 Flawed democracy	7.02 Flawed democracy	3.16 Authoritarian
United Nations Human Development Index[b] Ranking (score) out of 189 countries	185 (.433)	153 (.563)	162 (.538)	88 (.756)	138 (.611)	101 (.734)	150 (.571)
Poverty rate (World Bank)	64.9%	37.5%	39.5%	21%	23.4%	19.9%	38.3%

The Democracy Index uses 60 indicators grouped in five categories, measuring pluralism, civil liberties, and political culture. Full democracies = 8.01–10; flawed democracies = 6.01–7; hybrid regimes = 4.01–6; authoritarian regimes = 0–4. The Democracy Index is compiled by the Economist Intelligence Unit, a research division of the Economist Group, the private company which publishes the weekly newspaper, *The Economist*.

The Human Development Index is compiled by the United Nations. The metric quantifies achievements across three broad domains, one measuring health and longevity, one measuring knowledge, and the third measuring standard of living. Data for 2019 are presented.

4

Becoming a Learning Community

Oakland, California, May 9, 2018

Trains run through Jack London Square long before dawn, shaking the floors and walls of the harborside buildings as they rumble past. The vibrating bass of a train's engine wakes me (Robin) long before the chirping bird sounds of my cellphone's alarm clock swell to crescendo. I search in the dark for my laptop on the bedside table. I flip open the cover. I press the power on. The screen glows blue and then transforms into a photograph of a faraway coast. I review my notes for the day's meetings. I dial home. I kill time. I stand on the tiny balcony of my hotel room overlooking the harbor. Bursts and flashes of gold glimmer on the murky water as the sun ascends. The 6:45 a.m. ferry to San Francisco fills with commuters. Time to shower and dress. After a quick cup of coffee in the hotel's empty bar, I pull on my jacket, sling my backpack over my shoulders, and head uphill.

The walk from Jack London Square up Broadway should take me 15 minutes. Twelve at a rapid pace. I leave the Waterfront in plenty of time. I scamper across the tracks that run along Embarcadero West. It is just after 8 a.m. I pass a man tucked into the entryway just short of the Slàinte Irish Pub on the corner of 2nd Street. He snores gently on the tattered remnants of a cardboard box in a grime-stained sleeping bag. His terrier eyes me from where she naps, nestled in his mane of chestnut curls. At every street corner and in every vestibule, someone reclines in a makeshift bed constructed of salvaged material placed on cold cement ground. Near Buttercup, just beyond Souley Vegan, and in the city of tents lining the underpass of the Nimitz and John B. Williams Freeways. I stride right past 11th Street and the Bart Station entrance before realizing the numbers are running the wrong way. I head back to 11th. I gaze up at the shell of a grand old brick office tower under construction. I check my phone. This is the address in the email. I march toward 12th again. I tuck my head into the lobby of a building at an address printed on the back of an old MPact report. The man attending to the front desk remembers them. He points me down the street. The WeWork building at 1111 Broadway, he instructs.

I have come to Oakland to meet the MPact team for the first time. This is the first test of how George's colleagues receive my presence. I have taken similar tests before, but my anxieties are provoked each time I embark on a new partnership. Passing an initial test of trustworthiness and sincerity in one circumstance is no guarantee of passing that test in another. It is a critical test. Why are you here? Why do you care about us? Are you an ally or a threat? I have been posed these questions indirectly

Breaking Barriers. Robin Lin Miller and George Ayala, Oxford University Press. © Oxford University Press 2024.
DOI: 10.1093/oso/9780197647684.003.0005

(and directly) on more than one occasion. I have learned to breathe through the over-whelming sense of vulnerability induced by these queries and meet them head-on. The greater vulnerability is not mine. It belongs to those who are wary of evalua-tors and especially to those who have not yet learned that wariness might be wise. Evaluation, like any other form of social inquiry, may not always be performed with the interests of communities in mind.

I have also flown to Oakland to take initial stock of how, if at all, monitoring and evaluation inform MPact's work. MPact is an evidence-driven activist organization with a modest internal research function, but in our conversations over the prior 2 years, George has identified evaluation as an area ripe for growth. He has been plain that most of what MPact is typically asked to do by its funders is not evaluation, but a form of accountability monitoring that strikes him as a burdensome administra-tive chore. Not useful in the least. Monitoring is never intended for MPact's ben-efit. Nor is it responsive to the nature of its work. It is a hollow exercise to keep the lights on. Evaluation, though it holds the promise of being useful, is an unaffordable luxury. Funders' expectations for evaluation are unrealistic anyway and, in the HIV arena, too often "researchy" efforts grounded in an experimental methodological fundamentalism that makes little sense for small community-led organizations like MPact. Helping MPact land on sensible evaluation strategies is among my newfound responsibilities.

In this chapter, I describe the process of establishing my relationship with the members of the MPact team who worked on Project ACT. Every act of community engagement, whether as an evaluator or community researcher, demands intense self-examination and substantial preparation as its starting point. I illustrate how I built a trusting and reciprocal relationship with the MPact team members, and later, the entire Project ACT team—a relationship that permitted us to explore our mu-tual interests and needs, center our shared humanity and community commitment, and pave the foundation for the evaluation of Project ACT. I will show why flexibility and adaptation are necessary to pave the way for evaluating community-led organi-zational activities.

George's observations about and experiences of monitoring and evaluation come to me as no surprise. Evaluation is often under-capacitated and poorly resourced in organizations like his (Carman, 2007, 2011; Carman & Fredericks, 2010). The do-mestic evaluation literature documents the perception that expectations for moni-toring and evaluation seldom align with what community actors value, want, need, or do. The international literature echoes North American refrains. As powerfully illustrated in Robert Lorway's ethnographic account of a sex worker–led initiative in India, accountability-focused monitoring and evaluation can transform crea-tive, vibrant community-led outreach endeavors into intrusive, corporatized activ-ities (Lorway, 2017, pp. 100–101). The tyranny of some monitoring and evaluation activities in international settings is arguably worse because too often the guiding values and standards originate in the Global North and are imposed on actors from the Global South (Chilisa & Mertens, 2021), perpetuating colonial dynamics (see

Chapter 2). An ethnographic study by Matthew Thomann describes this dynamic well. Thomann documents the effects of a large North American implementing partner of PEPFAR on several small community-led organizations that provide safe havens for LGBT people in the deeply hostile environment of Côte d'Ivoire.[1] In his recounting, the implementing partner imposed a performance-based pay model for community outreach on the community-led organizations. Thomann writes:

> As subcontractors in this system, HIV peer educators and activists are charged with doing the "on the ground" work of reaching MSM, while staff at Heartland engage in monitoring and programme evaluation and conduct financial audits that carry with them the threat of funding cuts. In our discussions about their relationships with foreign donors and intermediary NGOs, peer educators and activists at Alternative and Arc-en-Ciel complained of a relentless focus on numbers-based results. Taped to the wall of Claver's office were poster-board sized post-Its with "new MSM" targets to be reached that year. These numbers were a constant source of anxiety and frustration for the staff at Alternative. In 2011, Heartland set the target at 1570 MSM reached. In 2012, the target jumped to 2153 new MSM. The staff often joked about the enormity of these targets, noting that if targets continued to rise this way in 2013, they would have to start "making MSM." (Thomann, 2016, p. 1004)[2]

This results-based pay-for-performance system stripped long-term social and material support from the organizations' constituents and threatened to undermine their community relationships. When I visit Alternative Côte d'Ivoire 6 years after Thomann, I find 20" × 23" sticky notes inscribed with columns of tick marks pasted to the walls, attesting to enduring pressure to ensure its financial survival by counting HIV-testing encounters with newly minted men.

In a world tilted hard toward evidence-based programs readily amenable to "conventional" evaluation and one in which support for advocacy is increasingly difficult to secure, George wished for an evaluation approach that might make a better case for activists' contributions to societal change. He longed for evaluations that supported rather than undermined or limited his efforts. George genuinely desired widespread evaluation of MPact's advocacy work for more reasons than simply to show its value. He wanted MPact to do what it does better and for its staff to have new ways to learn and share with other activists. Embedding myself in the organization for a year to support his ambitions and enhance my own learning about advocacy evaluation might provide us each a rare opportunity.

The Difficult Terrain of Evaluating Advocacy

Scholarship on advocacy evaluation grew sharply over the 2 decades leading up to my arrival at MPact. Advocacy, as defined in this literature, broadly refers to organized efforts by citizens to apply pressure on the societal institutions that protect the status quo and preserve unequal access to power. These pillars might be civic, commercial, judicial, or political. Advocacy efforts place pressure on society's duty bearers—the entities and individuals obligated to realize rights—to change the social policies and institutional practices that maintain inequity. Advocacy may involve a wide array of strategies and tactics—from birddogging officials[3] to organizing public protests to providing testimony to launching media campaigns to orchestrating petition drives. The model of advocacy MPact observes reflects the philosophy and strategies articulated by Saul Alinsky (1989). Alinsky anchored his approach to policy and social change in collective action, uniting community members to address the shared problems that affect their lives. Alinsky relied on an arsenal of core tactics that include building awareness, mobilizing citizens, cultivating community capacity, and conducting action research and policy analysis (Alinsky, 1989; Beckerman, 2022a, 2022b). MPact adheres to a similar tactical model, as George lays out in the previous chapter. MPact convenes its network of partners across the world, brokers their connections, bolsters their skills, and engages in direct policy advocacy rooted in empirical research and policy analysis.

Evaluators who write on advocacy evaluation are persuasive that the assumptions underlying many traditional methods and approaches to practice do not suit advocacy at all. As Barbara Klugman recently observed:

> I've learnt that when hiring a staff member to support social justice groups in data-gathering, documenting, and making sense of their efforts, they need to be wary of applicants whose only experience in "M&E" is checklist monitoring of compliance to contracts for funder-supported service provision, where data is not used for evaluation. They should rather seek someone who has experience in activism and advocacy with training in social or political theory, who will bring to bear the principle of collective action, and an evaluative lens. (Klugman, 2022)

Advocacy evaluation, as Klugman argues, demands that one fuse evaluative thinking (Buckley et al., 2015; Schwandt, 2015, 2018; Vo & Archibald, 2018) with advocacy's dynamism and an unwavering commitment to social justice.

Advocacy presents evaluators with thorny problems due to its ambiguous and uncertain nature. It is unlike the programs that most evaluators train to study. Evaluation textbooks typically highlight programs that authors such as Michael Quinn Patton and Patricia Rogers label as "simple" in their complexity (see, for example, Patton & Campbell-Patton, 2022). Simple programs are stable and routine in how they operate over time, linear in their logic, and especially in the context of the evidence-based practice movement, manualized or scripted. Advocacy, by contrast, is an undertaking that by necessity shifts and turns in nonrecurring, unpredictable, and unforeseen directions. The boundaries of a specific advocacy effort can enlarge and contract unpredictably as opportunities and leverage points open and close or the environment changes. Agility and the rapid replacement of an initial plan with alternatives is the name of the game.

A textbook program possesses outcomes that are identifiable at the start, occurring within a narrow range of possibilities and over a foreseeable timescale. Advocacy outcomes, by contrast, are difficult to anticipate in nature and timing (Arensman, 2020; Arensman & Van Wessel, 2018; Teles & Schmitt, 2011). It may take years of advocacy effort before even small wins are discernable and activists gain traction. A textbook program possesses personnel and activity boundaries that can often be determined with acceptable, albeit imperfect, certainty. Advocacy's actors change as alliances are forged and dissolved and as new champions and opponents emerge. In textbook programs, routine failure and chronic blowback are not ordinary expectations. It is typical in advocacy to endure setbacks and suffer defeat, if for no other reason than advocacy, by its nature, is an encounter with forceful opposition. For all these reasons and more, advocacy evaluation requires a distinctive logic and specialized techniques appropriate to complex, dynamic endeavors.

Unsurprisingly, advocacy evaluators draw heavily on approaches stemming from the causal logics of narration and contribution rather than from the attributional logic undergirding experimentation and quasi-experimentation.[4] Advocacy evaluators favor designs that are nimble, flexible, and iterative. They apply techniques that are engaged, calling upon agile tools that are designed specifically to encourage a reflective advocacy practice, such as intense period debriefs, critical incident timelines, and media tracking (Coffman & Reed, 2009; Coffman, no date; Gardner & Brindis, 2017; Innovation Network, 2007; Raynor et al., 2021).[5] Advocacy evaluators prefer shedding light on the process of advocating and real-time learning from confrontations with power (Klugman, 2022; Schlangen & Coe, 2021). In this approach, the evaluator is an ally and support resource to activists.

Evaluating Human Rights Advocacy

Despite the richness of discussion among policy and advocacy evaluators about how to build sound evidence through approaches that are fit to task, the evolving canon omits robust guidance on evaluating: in the Global South, in nondemocratic settings, in the context of authoritarian regimes, on behalf of sexual and gender minority people, and in countries criminalizing same-sex sexual interaction (Esala et al., 2022; Miller, 2021; Miller & Tohme, 2022). The challenges of evaluating human rights advocacy closely overlap those of other forms of advocacy, but not entirely. A handful of writers have taken up the special issues human rights advocacy presents (e.g., Esala et al., 2022; Klugman, 2011; Schlangen, 2014). Rhonda Schlangen, for example, notes that the worth of human rights advocacy is moral, suggesting entirely different indicators of its value than commonly observed elsewhere in evaluation. The kinds of activities engaged in by human rights champions cannot always be judged on their outcomes or reflected by simple indicators. The human rights lawyer may not succeed in freeing a client from prison, Schlangen observes, but from a human rights perspective, they ought to persist in trying. Repeated failure, she argues, does not have the same implications or meaning as it might for other endeavors.

Human rights advocacy differs from other types of advocacy work in that it is especially dangerous (see Chapters 1 and 2). In some contexts, engaging in human rights advocacy is treasonous. Human rights activists (and evaluators working with them) bear heightened risks that include digital and physical surveillance, violence, torture, and detention. Activists may operate in cells for the protection of their movement and its members. Evaluators may never know, nor should they know, the entire story of how some activists' networks function because of the potential to damage their movements (Brodsky, 2003; Brodsky & Faryal, 2006). Paper records may be undesirable because of the risk of harm they pose in the wrong hands. Digital security of data is paramount, yet difficult to ensure. These are among the special considerations that human rights advocacy evaluators must also manage, so as not to undermine human rights movements or jeopardize the security of activists.

A recent review of the human rights advocacy evaluation literature in the Global South (Esala at al., 2022) affirms that when the MPact team and I began to work together, an especially limited base of evaluation literature was available to draw on for wisdom pertinent to African and Caribbean contexts, the key regions of focus during our collaboration. Instead, the robust, emerging literature on practice originated principally from evaluations of policy advocacy in constitutional democracies and in Global North settings. This is still the case. Writing on human rights advocacy evaluation remains a largely grey literature generated by North Americans and Western Europeans. This literature does not appear to address evaluations of sexual and gender minority rights initiatives in the Global South at all. Insights into how community-led organizations pursue human rights issues for sexual and minority people is terrain principally covered by a small number of journalists, activist-practitioner scholars, sociologists, and anthropologists, most of whom move in separate disciplinary circles and scholarly communities of practice from evaluators. Phillips and colleagues (2022) point to wide variation across time and place in the social and political support of sexual and gender minority people. Understanding the historical and present-day ways in which oppression shapes sexual and gender minority experiences in specific times and places, assists evaluators to ensure their work serves local political aims and does not inadvertently reinforce local oppressions (Corey-Boulet, 2019). From this standpoint, the lack of guidance on evaluating sexual and gender minority human rights advocacy in the geopolitical context of Africa and the Caribbean is vexing.

These are among the gaps, complexities, and unknowns playing over and over in my mind as I stride up and down Broadway in the crisp May morning air, passing my destination time and again. I spy the WeWork building. I enter the lobby. Nadia Rafif, MPact's director of policy, is waiting. She greets me warmly. We ride the elevator to the fifth floor. As I step into the WeWork common space, I do not anticipate that MPact's newest effort, Project ACT, will become my sole preoccupation for the next 2.5 years.

Staff gradually arrive, passing through the common area to dump their bags in the single 12' × 20' office the 13 staff share. They seldom have occasion to appreciate its spectacular northward and westward views of the city. They are constantly on the road. Today is a rare homecoming. Nadia and I head downstairs, balancing coffee mugs on laptops. Others soon follow. George. Greg. Omar. Stephen. Johnny. We wedge ourselves into a small, dimly lit conference room on the third floor. The team members introduce themselves. Stephen shifts in his seat. He asks, "Why do you care about gay men?" My stomach knots. I acknowledge the significance of his question and thank him for asking it. The personal bridges I have traversed connecting me to the work I have chosen to do throughout my career are sturdy bridges to collaboration with MPact. They connect me to the work we will do together in profoundly personal, deeply emotional, and psychologically complicated ways. I share pieces of myself. Fire Island. GMHC. I speak about the world I want to live in. George adds that he and I have known each other for over 30 years. He appreciates how I think about evaluation and how I do it. He trusts me to navigate MPact's waters. Stephen expresses his reluctant reassurance.

We move on. Nadia and the team offer me an overview of MPact's current projects and activities. I ask how monitoring and evaluation inform the various projects, which, as it turns out, is little if at all. The staff affirm what George forewarned. A sort of death by monitoring has been their most common experience. Almost to a person, everyone has suffered from monitoring strategies that offered them little value in return for the effort they required. I ask them to reflect on a time when they have been part of an evaluation process that succeeded in providing them with useful insights to improve their effort, enhance their advocacy influence, or convey the value of what they do. No one save Stephen can point to an evaluation experience that possesses these characteristics. The staff create logic models and theories of change for themselves as visual reminders of their aspirations. They meet funders' accountability requirements. I ask what they hope for in an evaluation framework. A realistic approach to evaluating advocacy. An evaluation approach that supports their learning. An evaluation approach that clarifies the contribution they make to their partners' growth and to their partner's advocacy successes. As we are about to conclude our morning discussion, George leans slightly forward in his chair. He has an idea: Why don't you evaluate the new project, Project ACT? That might be the ideal way to contribute evaluation advice to his team, develop a framework for MPact to carry into its future, and simultaneously meet my learning objectives. I pause. I know a little bit about Project ACT. I know it is huge in its scope and ambition. I know it will engage activists across multiple countries. I know its details remain unknown. I know its evaluation considerations are dizzying to contemplate, even absent its vagueness. I say "yes."

We pile into the elevator and head over to Clay Street for lunch. We devote the afternoon to launch plans for Project ACT. To inaugurate Project ACT, we will host a 3-day project kick-off retreat. We have less than 4 weeks to prepare. We design the retreat to provide an occasion for team building, for defining and refining the advocacy plans, and for agreeing on a monitoring and evaluation framework. We sketch out a preliminary retreat agenda to ensure that each partner settles on a strategy and tactics that are robust yet realistic. Our discussion is fast moving. Elements of the agenda quickly emerge and are divvied up among us to flesh out. Although we had intended to devote time to the evaluation's planning, the urgency of preparing for the retreat consumes our time. I leave Oakland the following morning with evaluation decisions postponed to the future. We have only 23 months left to show the Elton John AIDS Foundation that their modest investment in advocacy will pay off.

Siem Reap, Cambodia, June 5–8, 2018

I land in Siem Reap[6] on a near empty flight out of Shanghai just after 10 p.m. on Tuesday, June 5, the night before the retreat is to start. By 11 p.m. my tuk-tuk is speeding along the short distance from the airport toward National Road 6 and the Angkor Paradise Hotel. Although it is long after dark, the day's heat still hangs in the air like a dense cloud of steam. I settle myself in a teak-walled room on the second floor of the hotel just after midnight. I text home before climbing into an ornately carved bed. I must sleep, but my body remains confident it is truly midday. I doze fitfully for the next 3 hours. I rise to join some of the MPact team for breakfast before heading to the meeting room where we, 14 of the activists who will lead the work on the ground, and two translators will spend the next 3 days collectively refining the plans of attack on stigma, discrimination, and violence.

Day One: Focusing

A verdant garden dense with palm trees, fragrant rumduols, and trellised orchids encircles the outdoor pool. I walk alongside its edge to reach the stairs leading up to our second-floor meeting room. Sweat forms on my forehead as I climb to the second level. I pass through an air-conditioned foyer and a second set of doors leading into our meeting space. The temperature indoors is bracing in contrast to the morning's heat. Greg, MPact's communications specialist and a member of our Project ACT Team, and Johnny sit just inside the door at a table littered with equipment and supplies. "Sign in over here, Robin." Johnny points to a sheet on the table.

The room is set with four round tables. A large banner covers the far wall announcing the launch of Project ACT. A projection screen stands just in front of the banner. Our partners claim places at the tables. Nadia moves about the room, her camera in hand, taking photographs and greeting our colleagues. "Bonjour! Ça va?" she calls out excitedly, embracing Guy, then Emil, activists from Cameroon, as they find their way to a table. Guy, Emil, and their translator, Chantal, are soon joined by other Francophone activists, Claude and Abou from Côte d'Ivoire and Pierre from Burundi. Omar perches on a chair at the front of the room chatting in rapid-fire

Spanish with the Dominicans, Miguel and Isabella, and their translator, Louis. They speak with such speed I hardly catch a word. Penya and Mandla from Zimbabwe, Kofi and Michael from Ghana, Prosper from Burundi, and Akoni and Jaden from Jamaica claim open spots at the tables. I join Mohan and Stephen. I pull out my laptop, pens, and the thick pads of paper I will use to record field notes of the meeting. Mohan smiles as he eyes my stockpile. Stephen leans forward.

"Ready?"
"Yes, let's go."

Mohan and I respond in unison. Stephen stands and moves to the front of the room.

The agenda will alternate between activities created to solidify our camaraderie and activities to support our ability to leave Cambodia with solid and focused advocacy workplans. The MPact team members will rotate through the role of facilitator, and partners will lead us through short team-building exercises and activities to boost our energy level. Johnny and Greg set the stage for these energizing activities with one in which we create Facebook profiles on cards, which Greg posts in a line on the wall as we each complete them. At Johnny's instruction, we survey the profiles, charged with matching intriguing profiles to their owner. As each person is matched to their drawing, they must speak about it. Prosper stands before the card on which he drew the shape of the Twitter bird. He explains that Twitter is a safe place to talk about what he loves and to find community. Guy drew a planet. Underneath his planet he wrote: "Dreaming that the future will be more perfect." Living on another planet, he explains, might offer the opportunity to meet people who are more tolerant than those he encounters on earth. Throughout the meeting, we post messages to one another, as we might on social media. By mid-morning, Penya receives a message appreciating her contagious smile and joyful spirit. The anonymous note urges Penya: "Keep on."

Each country team briefly presents their initial ideas for the advocacy work they desire to pursue, beginning with their assessment of local barriers to health care. Akoni begins. He indicates that in Jamaica stigma and discrimination are pervasive in arenas of life that enable health and facilitate LGBT people's willingness to access the country's system of socialized medicine. Homophobic violence, housing insecurity, and unemployment top the list. In Cameroon, Emil says that the criminalization law and health care providers' beliefs and values conflict with the medical code of ethics to provide care to all. Providers cave to their prejudices, refusing services and humiliating patients who are brave enough (or sick enough) to pursue care. Miguel shares that Dominican clinical staff are woefully unprepared to offer care that is affirming and likely to retain people. Affirming care is difficult to locate in Ghana, too, offers Kofi, and fear of accessing it is compounded by widespread discrimination and extortion. Prosper observes Burundians lack systems to document and report human rights violations. There is no advocacy network infrastructure to speak of. Even gathering five people together is forbidden, hampering mobilization efforts. Claude notes that in Côte d'Ivoire, mainstream media outlets portray gay men and the issues surrounding their HIV-related medical needs in damaging ways. Reportage labels competent and friendly health care clinics as "gay," antagonizing their staffs and causing attendance to decline for fear of stigmatization and violence. In Zimbabwe, Penya observes, gay men receive poor care that rarely aligns with the country's patient charter of rights. As each team presents, they lay out a general plan of attack to address these pervasive problems.

The MPact team occasionally poses questions to presenting teams, pushing them to begin to identify feasible and specific advocacy actions that can be mounted to address these high-priority barriers to care. Others jump in, calling on their peers to provide clarity on their nascent ideas. When we break for lunch, the MPact team and I debrief. The initial ideas lack necessary specificity. They are not realistic. Concepts such as "empowerment" and "affirming care" require concise operationalization. Advocacy needs to move to the center. We adjust our approach to the afternoon's agenda. We want to ensure partners understand that they must use this retreat to revise their plans to craft novel and feasible advocacy efforts that are consistent with the aims of Project ACT.

Johnny guides us through an exercise to foster esprit de corps, after which Omar leads the group through an advocacy case study. The case, set in Malawi, concerns a gay couple who were imprisoned and subsequently released by presidential order. The group dissects the case, identifying the advocacy targets, tactics, champions, and obstacles to success in obtaining the men's release. Tear sheets fill with lists. Omar prompts the group to identify the positive effects of the advocacy. People name the public discussion that the advocacy generated about gay men and their rights. They cite the men's ultimate release. They point to the increased profile of the issues in national debate. "What about the negatives?" Omar queries, pointing out that planning for negative impacts is important. Another list rapidly develops. The fear and risk of violence to the men. The colonizing narrative of Western intervention. Affirming the promotion of Western immorality. The role of the West in demotivating local activists. Partners work in teams to craft definitions of advocacy to guide their work: speaking up, drawing a community's attention to critical issues, and directing decision makers toward a solution. Omar wraps up the session. In 2 years, people will not be able to accomplish a lot of what they want to do. Johnny jumps in. "Advocacy is about the process." Omar calls for a volunteer to close the session. We sing together in a call-and-response.

Stephen divides participants into groups. He instructs them to identify ten steps in advocacy and put them in order. I watch Kofi write out steps in red marker as Mandla rearranges them on an easel in consultation with the other members of his group. They produce a praise-winning list: problem identification, problem clarification analysis, research on the issue, defining change, selecting a target audience, identifying allies, selecting a medium, taking action, documenting action, celebrating, and restrategizing. They indicate evaluation and resource mobilization are ongoing activities necessary to support action. We discuss the need to celebrate wins and publicize them, leading to the insight that advocacy is not necessarily about being the one who gets credit. I underline this in my notes. The belief in collective wins made possible through the contribution of many actors resonates with the contribution-oriented evaluation strategies I have been studying. I take note, too, that only Mandla's and Kofi's team mentioned evaluation is an ongoing aspect of advocacy.

We play a quick game. Omar begins. He tells us it is a rainy day. He is going to pass to someone in the group who must state a consequence of the fact it is raining. The next person in the chain must identify a consequence in turn. Rain causes a traffic jam. People are late for work. People lose their jobs. People stumble to identify effects at first. Causes and effects are occasionally peculiar, as they are translated to Spanish and French and back again. Consequences and effects loop back on one another. Parents beg in the streets. There is a traffic jam. We laugh, stop, reverse. Omar offers that people do get stuck conducting problem analyses. They might move in circles. We move forward again.

Omar tells the group that a concise problem statement identifies the proximal and root causes of a problem and its immediate and distal effects. He offers the metaphor of a tree. He stands before an easel at the front of the room, sketching a tree. Its roots travel deep into the soil. Its branches rise high above its trunk. He provides examples of specific, clear problem statements. He passes out large sheets of paper to each country team, instructing them to revise their project problem statement and map out causes and effects. "Revise what you are thinking about," he counsels, "because there is strategic and practical value in focusing on just one well-specified problem." Teams lean over their sheets of paper, drawing trunks, roots, and branches. Country leads join their partners, probing for causes and effects. When the statements are shared, the MPact staff note their promise. They point to the need for further revision. Assumptions must be reasonable, they say, and focused on a single problem. Statements must be concrete, with clear distinctions between root and proximal causes and intermediate and distal effects. It is late. We must finish this activity in the morning. The problem statements are too important not to get right. We form a circle. We toss our meeting mascot, Polly the Pride Bear, from one person to the next. As we hold Polly in our hands, we offer one word to describe how we feel. Nervous. Excited. Eager. Enlightened. Grateful.

The MPact team and I gather to debrief. We are pleased by the strong and positive group dynamics. We are eager to craft a cohesive, coherent multicountry project. To help partners step out of their history. To assist them to chart a realistic timeline of what they are likely to accomplish. We cannot move forward without solid problem statements and root cause analyses. We rearrange tomorrow's agenda. We drop, shorten, and push items to another day. They depart in preparation for an exceptional group dinner, an authentic Khmer meal and classical dance performance at a neighborhood pavilion. I stay behind, photographing the sticky notes and other items blanketing the room's walls, arriving in the lobby just in time to join the departing group.

Day Two: Power

We file into the meeting room, its walls crowded with the paper remnants of yesterday's effort. We silently write our hopes on small Post-it® paper, which Nadia collects. We hope to learn from each other. We hope to continue building our relationships with each other. We hope to challenge each other. We hope to improve our skills in developing workplans. We hope for enlightenment. We hope to attain excellence in advocacy. We continue reviewing problem statements. The MPact staff are increasingly pointed in their feedback. They ask for evidence informing the problem statements. They ask about policies and structures and accountability. They push for articulation of the causes of problems. They point to advocacy opportunities. They challenge the logic of cause-effect connections. As the discussion proceeds, country teams attend closely. They bend their heads over the papers spread before them, whispering back and forth, a signal they understand how deeply they must revise.

Stephen instructs the teams on how to prepare a target map. He reminds the teams they are focused on complex problems with unique local histories. Drawing the stakeholders and their relationships to one another, he says, will permit you to see who you can leverage and what relationships you ought to change or to create. Changing and establishing relationships, he observes, is a fundamental aspect of advocacy. Stephen illustrates his point by sketching a stick-figure man and a stick-figure nurse, who discriminates against the man. The two are connected through their patient–provider interaction. He draws the nurse's connections to other professionals and units within the hierarchical structure of staffing in a hospital. He draws the man's connections within the relational structure of his community. The country teams develop their own maps, enumerating local relationships with the guidance and input of MPact staff. Stephen instructs.

> "Look at your maps. Identify the people in the chain with decision-making power or more power than others in the relationship chains."
>
> "What do you mean by power?" Kofi calls out.
>
> Stephen responds, "Power is manifested in control of material and human resources, authority, knowledge, and expertise."
>
> Mandla presses, "What are the signs of community power?"

Stephen offers that a community's power could be suggested by its size, relationships, authority, resources, skills, values, or ideology. Stephen displays a slide on the projection screen defining people with power as those who enjoy the support of society's pillars such as police, schools, religious institutions, media, commerce, government, and systems of care. The teams return to their power analysis. For each stakeholder who holds power, they list what the stakeholder is likely to believe about the problem and issues. They indicate the values that might motivate the stakeholder. They identify how the stakeholder makes decisions. They draw the ties that connect the stakeholder to others, tracing webs of relationships, until they hit on connections that trace back to themselves.

We take a break for lunch, during which we adjust our agenda again. When we resume, Mandla leads us through a rousing energizer to beat the postlunch slump of the sweltering Cambodian afternoon. We raise our right arms above our heads. We count aloud to seven, shaking our hands in the air. We raise our left hand next, counting aloud to seven again. We kick seven times with our right foot, then seven times with our left, shouting the numbers aloud. We count to six, then five, then four, then three, then two, then one. We leap into the air, shouting "MPact!" in unison.

The teams present their stakeholder maps and power analyses. The exercise succeeded! Teams identified high-level targets who possess the power to change systems or hold them to account. Strategic targets are coming into view. National human rights commissions lack a clear relationship to LGBT communities but are well positioned to influence country-level change. There are new commissioners. That is a window of opportunity. Ah ha! The push must be up and down simultaneously; upward from the street-level bureaucracies that are closest to providers and downward from ministers who may not be aware of the issues but aspire to be good social stewards. Systems of redress must be strengthened. Editors must be targeted. Relationships must be cultivated between media and public health country coordinating mechanisms. Teams are now focused on points of leverage in the chain of power. We celebrate by playing telephone. "Nadia wears red boots on rainy days but not on Mondays and Tuesdays" sails down the line to the final person, who exclaims "On Mondays and Tuesdays, I am pregnant." We erupt into fits of laughter.

Stephen presents the concept of a theory of change, the if-then logic of event sequences and key assumptions. Country teams sketch theories of change for critique. But we are past schedule. We must dismiss the group for the day. The walls are now covered. Cross-fertilization is occurring. We are happy to see it. But we moved too quickly through critical exercises. Concepts must meet the threshold for signing a contract. We toss out the agenda for our final day. Our time will go to revising and presenting revised plans for Project ACT. Weary, we head out in small groups to explore the local drag scene.

Day Three: A Vision for Advocacy

In the morning, we begin by posting new learnings, observations, and hopes on the wall. I study the pieces of paper, reading the notes of appreciation for key learnings about workplan development and the finer points of advocacy. Notes celebrate the positive spirit in the room, the cross-fertilization, and the constructive criticism. Notes express relief at not being alone. Notes convey excitement at an emerging collective vision.

We attend briefly to business and touch on the agenda items we must drop. The evaluation is one. I share that we will use evaluation as learning space and that we will design the evaluation collaboratively. I request volunteers to work with me, Johnny, and Mohan on creating our plan. Abou, Claude, Pierre, and Emil raise their hands. Greg quickly reviews tips on communication strategy, followed by Mohan leading us through a rapid discussion of safety and security. He encourages teams to plan and budget for safety and security, including the cost of safe meeting places that minimize exposing constituents to unnecessary risk. After all, he says, promoting safety and security is why Project ACT exists. We play a game. This time, we pretend we are the elements of a house. One after the other, we position our bodies in front of the banner, calling out what part of the house we represent, joining ourselves to the human pieces of the home already in place. A chimney stands. A window appears. Then a door. Someone lays flat on the floor, announcing they are the lawn. Another slides alongside him and pretends to be a pool. A tree rises from the edge of the lawn. A fence appears. Then flowers. Once our house is constructed, its magnificent lawn spread across the carpet of our meeting room, Greg requests that we stand together in front of the banner. In the photo he takes, we beam, fresh in the memory of the home we built together, each of us lending an essential piece to its construction. We break for lunch. The MPact team and I hang back to debrief. The morning felt too rushed. Typical.

When we reassemble, Johnny announces the teams will have 1 hour to work on revising their plan. He encourages tweaks, big and small.

"Maintain an open mind and heart to critiques," he recommends.
"Makes this an opportunity," Nadia urges.

The teams work intensely. Johnny lies on the floor next to Claude and Abou, as Claude sketches out a new plan for Côte d'Ivoire. Mohan, Penya, and Mandla lean over their draft plan for Zimbabwe, writing thoughts in marker as they confer. Omar, Stephen, Nadia, and I move among the remaining teams. An hour and 20 minutes pass. The teams want more time. We change the agenda again to allow the teams to keep flowing. At 3:30, Johnny calls time. He sets ground rules. Teams will present. Feedback will be offered. Teams may only offer clarification on points of confusion. Each team presents in turn. Plans are, in most cases, notably improved. We applaud progress. We gather in a circle, tossing Polly from one person to the next. As we catch Polly, we offer a reflection: we appreciate the expert facilitation, camaraderie, learning about advocacy and advocacy planning, the collaborative spirit, the opportunity to have input on things we usually have no say in such as evaluation, the supportive climate, the chance to understand what people in other countries are contending with. We are excited for what is to come.

Once the last of our partners turns in their evaluation and leaves the room, the MPact team and I huddle for a final time. After 3 intense days, we arrived in a place we did not anticipate. The meeting added value. Weaker projects would have been siloed without this retreat. We established rapport and trust. We are a learning community now. Although we will build the boat as we sail it, we have at least agreed to its raw materials. We turn our conversation to the weakest proposals, wondering if they are worth the risk. We must devise strategies to move these teams closer to an innovative advocacy vision. Our funders hope for momentous changes. Their expectations worry us. I pick my notes up off the table and stash them in my bag. I take one more round of photos of the sheets hanging on the walls before I step into the stifling moist heat of early evening. I tuck myself into a corner in the hotel's lobby and begin the lengthy process of elaborating my field notes of the meeting. When exhaustion eventually wins out, I head upstairs.

Amsterdam, Netherlands, July 22, 2018

The cavernous octagon marble hall in Amsterdam's KIT Royal Tropical Institute reverberates with the pulsating sounds of dance music. The techno drumbeat is audible from outside the historic neo-Renaissance brick and stone structure. Men gather in small groups on the building's grand stone steps, dragging on their cigarettes in time to the rhythmic pounding. I skirt clouds of smoke as I mount the stairs. Indoors, activists and a select group of the leading HIV-focused researchers from every corner of the world crowd the ornate entry hall. I make my way through the maze of pub tables ringed with people chewing muffins and sipping tea and coffee. Johnny dances across the floor. He grabs my hand. He leads me behind a black marble pillar accented with flourishes of gold to a hidden cache of t-shirts for MPact team members. Souvenir in hand, I wade back into the crowd.

This preconference meeting to the 2018 International AIDS Society conference kicks off an intense week of organizing and events for MPact. The staff has devoted nearly all their effort since we departed Cambodia to preparing this daylong preconference that spotlights community solutions to enhance the sexual health and rights of young gay and bisexual men. In addition, they have planned a satellite session, a networking zone, and events in the Global Village, mined the conference program to produce a comprehensive list of its offerings on gay and bisexual men's concerns, and scheduled a steady daily agenda of advocacy meetings for staff. The preparations were all consuming. Today's event includes two plenary panels and an afternoon of concurrent sessions. Twelve youth teams from Asia, Africa, the Caribbean, Latin America, and North America will workshop their innovations to improve sexual health. Experts have been recruited to coach youth teams through their final preparations. Youths' day will culminate in a pitch competition before this elite global audience to win US$10,000 in start-up support.

In Cambodia, the staff had warned me that turning their attention to planning the evaluation of Project ACT must wait until this preconference and the IAS conference were behind them. At most, they had said, they might be able to continue the process of refining the Project ACT workplans with the country teams. They hoped to sign a contract with each country's team by summer's end at the latest, depending upon how the workplans progressed. Coupling that effort with the preconference and IAS preparations would certainly overflow their plates. I was initially frustrated and puzzled that evaluation planning would be put on hold, not fully grasping the enormity of planning the preconference in addition to the week's long IAS schedule of events, sessions, and meetings.[7] I simply had no idea. It made sense to me once I climbed up the marble staircase leading into the Queen Maxima auditorium, took my seat, and started to thumb through the 23-page "Out with It!" program booklet.

My presence at the preconference was a deliberate move on the part of the Project ACT team. As one of the morning's panelists, I am tasked with encouraging the youth teams to build evaluative thinking into their plans and, ideally, actual evaluation activities. In so doing, I plan to establish a vision for evaluation that is likely to run counter to the vision held by many in the room. I came to Amsterdam ready to make my best case for the necessity and power of transformative evaluation. I climb onto the stage just after 11 a.m. In my remarks, I challenge the youth teams to help counter what I see as gross historical distortions in the base of evidence on HIV interventions, a distortion that arises from the fact that not everything worth evaluating earns that opportunity (Miller & Shinn, 2005; Rogers, 2016). What we know about promising interventions slants heavily toward intervention research studies designed in the hothouses of Global North universities, think tanks, and government centers and away from evaluations of community-designed and community-led solutions. Homegrown community solutions merit evaluation, too. Evaluation can help us to learn systematically from our missteps, trials, and triumphs. Evaluation and evaluative thinking are tools to help us. We can gain important insights on what it takes to do the work on the ground, day after day, year after year, in real-world circumstances when we invest time and effort in evaluation. If we are ever going to forge sustainable solutions to the HIV epidemic, we must use evaluation to learn from communities. We must be evaluative thinkers.

These are the same reasons I see the evaluation of Project ACT as so important. Over the weeks since leaving Cambodia, I have pored over MPact's annual reports, project case studies, and strategic planning documents. The Out with It! preconference reveals more about MPact and its values, people, stakeholders, and constituents than I had anticipated. MPact's values reflect deep sensitivity to the colonizing dynamics that might emerge from their base in the Global North and role in strengthening kindred organizations in the Global South. In my every interaction with MPact team members, they openly worry about how to operate in ways that respect and support local expertise. That is why in Project ACT they will not dictate what others must do. They will only establish loose parameters for using advocacy to attack impediments to accessing HIV care and will engage with country teams in the spirit of partnership. "I'm very sensitive about trying to tell people what to do because I've been on the opposite side. And I don't like it when global organizations or donors are trying to have me do their agenda as a Southerner," one explained when we chatted over Zoom. The very fact he works in a global organization in no way makes him more knowledgeable than those who work at country level: "I actually believe they know more than I do, because that's their environment. That's their work. And they know how the work is done."

Project ACT's complexities, its tremendous diversity—seven unique countries, each with their own histories, cultures, languages, Indigenous knowledge traditions, and colonial and postcolonial experiences—sits uncomfortably within the paradoxical dynamics of contemporary thinking on how evaluators ought to respond to the history of colonization. Made-in-Africa and Indigenous evaluation frameworks argue for elevating African and Indigenous experience and values over values imposed from cultural outsiders. These evaluation approaches aim to restore and preserve the African and Indigenous cultural norms and values devoured by colonization. As such, these movements are fundamentally emancipatory. They champion the fact that African and Indigenous values, lifeways, and worldviews are not necessarily akin to those of Global North actors. They recognize that what is idealized in the Global North may in fact be anomalous or even repulsive in the Global South. Sexual and gender minority human rights sit in the crosshairs of debates on what it means to be decolonizing.[8]

Current prescriptions for practice instruct evaluators to consider "how interventions in Africa contribute to realizing ideal communities on African terms" (Chilisa & Malunga, 2012, pages 37-38), but pose a dilemma for evaluations of efforts like Project ACT, at least in the sense that there are competing African visions for what is ideal. Local cultural values often labeled as African sometimes produce and maintain the very social inequities Project ACT critiques. Imperatives set down in guidance for evaluators state that evaluation stakeholders' cultural and religious beliefs must not be threatened (AfrEA, 2021). Project ACT will challenge and may threaten stakeholders' cultural and religious beliefs, a dynamic the evaluation might easily mirror. Indeed, if the evaluation is true to a transformative perspective (Mertens, 2009), in certain ways it must favor those who challenge prejudicial views, however gently. Is honoring justice and challenging oppression at odds with honoring African and Indigenous value systems? Can evaluators choose which African or Indigenous people's values to honor or which to dismiss? If so, how and on what basis? What are the consequences of the evaluator's choices for a decolonizing evaluation process? Evaluating Project ACT will beg these questions.

East Lansing, Michigan, September 12, 2018

Summer melts quickly away. Since arriving home from Amsterdam, we have begun planning the evaluation's details, described in About the Evaluation at the end of the book. Partners are inputting to the plan from afar. Most of the contracts are signed. Initial tranches have been wired. Advocacy has begun in several countries. We are almost ready to capture how advocacy works. We are truly underway.

PART III

ADVOCACY IN ACTION

We are like a person living in a house with multiple leaks. We run from place
to place and put our finger over each leak, then run to the next spot.

—**Johnny, MPact Country Lead**

The final part of this book, Chapters 5 through 9, describes how the activists in Project ACT pursued their advocacy agendas. We explore how activists strengthened the ability of sexual and gender minority constituencies to engage in advocacy actions and engaged allies to assist in their cause. We describe the challenges they overcame and their advocacy wins. We conclude this section with an examination of the principles of practice that enabled the success of the advocacy work and of the transnational partnership that supported these successes.

5

Promise Rises

Promise knew it would soon be his turn. He shifted in his seat, bumping his knee against the back of the white plastic chair in front of him as he pivoted his hips. The room, lit only by morning's winter light filtering through the open doorway and windows, was full; almost every one of the 32 plastics chairs that Mbuso and I had jammed together into barely discernable rows held someone. Promise sat quietly, speaking to no one, his face set in a sullen glare, his jaw clenched. Shifting again in his seat, he glanced up at the photos that lined the tops of the room's shadowed walls, the faces of his friends captured in elegant black-and-white portraits, daring the portrait artist to reveal their humanity in the camera's lens.

Mandla's voice called Promise to the only uncluttered floorspace at the front of the room. Couches. A flip chart. Overstuffed faux leather lounge chairs. Tables. LCD projector. Projector screen. Laptop. Footstools. These were all haphazardly shoved into a roughly 14' × 9' area at the front of the room to form the boundaries of a miniscule and cluttered makeshift stage. Promise rose. He pushed past knees pressed against the row of white plastic lawn chairs in front of his own. Stepping sidewise as best he could, he trained his eyes on the floor, moving carefully over bags and backpacks tucked between feet and chair legs. Once in the narrow aisle, he limped to the front of the room, past Mbuso leaning against the wall, past the matron perched on the edge of her wobbling chair, past Zandi and Thulani sharing a single leather lounge chair, Zandi perching on its arm. His right shoulder dipped with each step, his right leg dragging slightly behind, his foot incapable of rising much off the ground. His crown of twisted locks swayed as he walked, the top half of his body angling toward the wall, and then righting itself, like an inverted pendulum. When he reached the front of the room, he turned, lowered himself into the waiting chair, and lifted his angular face to address the crowd of nurses seated in rows before him. He sat, staring straight ahead, moving hardly at all, as Bunjiwe began to speak. He occasionally surveyed the nurses as she spoke, his eyes panning the room, measuring their reactions to her story. Then it was his turn.

He began slowly, in English at first, then in Ndebele, the language in which he could best express the resentment thundering through his lean frame. He told the nurses that he was a person living with HIV. He was also a gay man. He had been admitted to the local hospital in a seriously ill state. He spent his hospitalization in the men's ward, an open barrack-styled cavern typical of a 1950s-era tropical hospital. The ward contained about five or six rows of beds blanketed in blue, four beds to a row. Three or four on-duty nurses occupied a single desk set just inside the entrance

Breaking Barriers. Robin Lin Miller and George Ayala, Oxford University Press. © Oxford University Press 2024.
DOI: 10.1093/oso/9780197647684.003.0006

to the room. A communal bathroom was tucked behind a cement wall at the room's rear. Patients, visitors, and staff all freely roamed the crowded hall outside the open doorway. Promise's friends routinely visited him at lunchtime and in the early evenings, encircling his bed, as did the friends and families of the other men in his ward. Their presence punctuated each tedious bedridden day with moments of joy and glimmers of hope for his quick recovery.

Promise leaned forward abruptly. His hand, once draped over his knees, reached toward his audience, his palm upward. His rapid staccato accelerated. A nurse assigned to his ward took an instant dislike to him and especially to the presence of his friends. The routine gatherings of young queer men surrounding Promise's bed each day seemed to fill this nurse with disdain. Whenever the nurse passed by his bed or was required to attend to him, scorn tinged his face. Promise thought he once heard him spit "chomma"[1] under his breath as he passed alongside Promise's bed. One afternoon, the nurse came to Promise's bedside to administer his daily injection. Promise pointed to his bedside medication tray set on the opposite side of his bed from where the nurse stood. He reminded the nurse that his medication had already been administered that morning. The nurse ignored him, turning his back. He readied an injection from the nearest tray. Promise again asked why he was receiving an injection when one had already been administered. The nurse shot back in a growl that Promise should mind himself. Demons should not tell nurses what to do. Promise persisted to object while the nurse forcibly administered him an injection. It was only a few moments later, as the nurse began to enter the date and time record of the injection on Promise's medical card, that the nurse realized he had indeed injected Promise with a medication meant for the man in a nearby bed. But, by then, it was too late. Promise did not say what the neurotoxic medication was. He did not know. That did not matter to him. What did matter was that the medication error caused an acute drug-induced movement disorder that left Promise with partial paralysis and a pronounced permanent limp.

Promise abruptly ceased speaking. He shook visibly in his chair. He folded his arms over his chest, leaned back, and sat in a pained stony silence, staring straight ahead.

The nurses had initially attended to Promise with rapt attention. Now, they struggled to return his gaze, preferring to stare at the back of a chair or a page of the notebook balanced on a thigh or at the portraits of young people just like Promise lining the walls. They appeared startled by the realization that their hostile country environment fostered prejudices that made it so immensely difficult for a colleague to provide affirming care to Promise and made it even harder still for people like Promise to ever gain confidence in their care. Their eyes darted about the room, stricken looks on their faces. Perhaps Mandla would break the tension soon. Relieve their discomfort. Console them.

Promise shared his profoundly troubling experience of interpersonal stigma and its personal impact as part of a health care worker sensitization training that I (Robin) witnessed on a cool and cloudless Saturday morning in Bulawayo, Zimbabwe, in July 2019.[2] Health care worker sensitization was one component of an integrated set of

advocacy tactics pursued by the Sexual Rights Centre. In most Project ACT countries, preparing gay and bisexual men and transgender women to participate in social
action, as Promise did that morning, was foundational to the advocacy work they
conducted. Paths like the one Promise traversed to enable him to participate in advocacy tactics such as public speaking had to be paved for Project ACT to succeed. The
Project ACT partners had to counter the results of lifelong confrontations with prejudice and stigmatization on constituents by fostering a sense of agency and readiness
for action. In Burundi, Cameroon, Ghana, Jamaica, and Zimbabwe, constituents had
to be equipped to document discrimination in health care interactions. In Cameroon,
Côte d'Ivoire, Jamaica, and Zimbabwe, they had to be readied to provide testimony
on blatant acts of discrimination, humiliation, and violence during trainings and in
mainstream and social media. In Jamaica and Zimbabwe, they had to be supported
to take on new leadership roles and, with these roles, greater visibility. In Ghana,
Jamaica, and Zimbabwe, they had to be primed to claim their rights in health care
and other settings. The partners who took on the challenge of preparing constituents
to engage in advocacy actions did so in varied ways. This chapter describes how the
Project ACT partners prepared their constituents to contribute to local advocacy. We
focus on their tactical efforts to reduce internalized-stigma and promote confidence
in their constituents' political agency. We illustrate how healing and empowerment
guided their approaches.

Living Your Life Closed-Up

Models of empowerment suggest that before people can successfully mobilize for social change, they must harness a belief in their own agency and ability to act. Evaluator
Barbara Klugman refers to this as the "power within" (see also Starhawk, 1987). In her
conception, the ability to harness the power of a community—the power achieved
through mobilization, bonding, and creating linkages to sources of power—rests
on individuals' confidence they can be agents of change. To achieve power within,
people require opportunities to engage in concrete civic action, coupled with the so-
cialization experiences that build their emotional and relational competence and cement their bonds to others with whom they share common cause (Christens, 2021).
For LGBT people, building power within can include shedding deeply internalized
negative societal messages (Chapter 1; Pachankis & Jackson, 2022). For many of the
Project ACT partners, mechanisms to foster the development of healing and personal
growth proved an essential element of community mobilization.

   In many of the project countries, a principal obstacle to action derived from a
deeply rooted internalized or self-stigma,[3] resulting from living in stigmatizing contexts. Internalized stigma, as we discussed in Chapter 1, curbs help-seeking behaviors, reinforces social isolation, and exacerbates diverse health and mental health
disorders (Camp et al., 2020; Kane et al., 2019; National Academy of Sciences, 2020;
Sundararaj et al., 2021; UNAIDS, 2021f). Internalized stigma can manifest as denial,

fear of disclosure, identity concealment, and homonegativity. These manifestations of internalized stigma form the pathways by which structural and interpersonal stigma result in poor individual health and socioeconomic outcomes (Pachankis et al., 2021).

The effects of internalized stigma were readily apparent to the members of the Project ACT country teams. They routinely observed reluctance among constituents to claim their rights or take individual action to pursue societal change. A limited sense of personal agency, developed over years of encounters with stigmatization, often drove the hesitancy they observed. Akoni, for example, explained in one of our interviews that Jamaican health care workers regularly reported to him and other activists that internalized stigma was driving high rates of anxiety and depression, poor medication adherence, and reluctance to seek services among gay, bisexual, and transgender patients. The Jamaican Ministry of Health, through the National Family Planning Board's own research, had documented that internalized stigma was, in Akoni's words, "a huge impediment to reducing HIV prevalence among the population and ensuring that people get on treatment and stay on treatment." Yet he noted people who fund programs simply did not appreciate why internalized stigma was so urgent to address in an advocacy project. Addressing internalized stigma through Project ACT, he asserted, was catalytic in its potential:

> This is not simply about how the population access services, but how they just navigate spaces on a daily basis. So that a number of people that we interact with, the younger ones especially, recognize that their feeling of self impacts in a lot of ways on how they experience love, how they function at school, at work, and in even how they stand up to people who discriminate against them.

Dymond also asserted the significance of addressing internalized stigma as a precursor to community mobilization and to ensuring access to care:

> Because for a lot of them, they don't think of themselves as worthy of being treated fairly and treated in a humane way or even getting access to certain things, including health care. Because they thought themselves as dirty or they thought themselves as not being good or clean. Or not looking the way they should look or being the way they should be.

Jaden drove the point home when he reflected on the challenges of mobilizing people to pursue the community's rights. "People don't feel good enough about themselves to be advocates."

Structural and interpersonal stigma form a developmental backdrop for young sexual and gender minority people. Society inculcates normative heterosexist and gendered biases that sexual and gender minorities learn before they recognize these prejudices apply to them or learn how to overcome them (Pachankis & Jackson, 2022). For the Project ACT activists, ensuring that younger constituents developed positive self-regard in the face of structural stigma was a leading concern. Many wanted a different life for youth than they had experienced when they were teens and young adults. They also realized that generating demand for affirming services required their constituents to believe in their entitlement to humane and fair treatment. Eithan, a Jamaican advocate who worked closely with youth, noted that youth have "a lot of internalized homophobia," which he said is easy to notice from listening to what they say about themselves and about other sexual and gender minority people. Jamaican youth struggle, he said, with bullying from teachers and peers, which undermines their ability to come to terms with their identity in positive ways. Youth cannot depend on teachers and other adults in schools for support. They may even be targeted by these adults, which complicates the already arduous process of enduring peer harassment at school.

In a roundtable discussion of Jamaican teachers I observed, they described chronic abuses perpetuated by school administrators, teachers, and students in Jamaican schools, from primary school to university (Field note, September 21, 2019). They cited examples of hostile actions by school personnel, including a school administration's decision to eliminate the women's basketball program because it was believed to "produce lesbians," students in high school classrooms yelling "no fish!" when a peer they suspected of being gay raised their hands to respond to the teacher, and a tenured college professor who begins each of his classes with a prayer and lecture in which he asserts homosexuality is tantamount to the production of monsters. The teachers reported that school administrators prefer to move bullied youth to any school willing to take them, resulting in sexual and gender minority youth bouncing from one school to another without any guarantee of entering a less hostile setting, and losing academic ground in the meantime. The Jamaican youth I met described experiences of aggressive bullying and flagrant abuse by teachers, which led to the interruption of their educational progress and denied them opportunities that might provide an alternative means to secure belief in their self-worth.[4] These youth attributed their victimization in schools as a reaction to their gender expression being perceived as too effeminate, which the teachers affirmed.

In Zimbabwe, during July 2019, I met with 22 young gay and bisexual men in three small groups. The electricity was out for the first of what would prove to be a 4-day stretch, the government's strategy to slow its accumulating debts to neighboring countries for supplying it electric power. The Centre rarely used its generator to save its precious supply of diesel fuel, a commodity also in short, unpredictable supply and available only to those lucky enough to have access to US dollars. The men and I clustered together in a darkened room toward the rear of one of the Centre's walled compounds, leaving the window and door open to catch the morning's cross-breeze.

Our conversation focused on growing up as sexual minorities in Zimbabwe. The need to overcome self-hate and believe in one's self-worth was a prominent theme in each of my three conversations. "There is so much self-hate I grew up with," one young man said, as he spoke about why he valued the Centre and the efforts initiated as part of Project ACT. The others in the room nodded, then quickly added their personal reflections on experiencing internalized stigma. A similar conversation repeated itself in each of the remaining groups. "It was difficult to accept who I was," one young man offered. Another young man spoke of his need to "learn how to deal with" himself. "There is so much phobia in yourself," one added. The men agreed that dealing with self-hate requires a healing process.

Adult activists also shared life experiences and personal struggles weathering internalized stigma. One Cameroonian activist concluded the lifetime of insults, grievous family rejection, and financial abandonment he had suffered based on his sexual orientation are "a form of violence." There is no social safety net, he explained. Family is the center of life and essential to survival. He went on to describe how difficult it can be to realize one's potential after having suffered lifelong abuse and rejection. He mourned the numbers of young men he had met in his work who had internalized their self-loathing so deeply they could only sooth themselves through substance abuse. You live your life "closed-up," he observed, by which he meant you kept your traumatic experiences and emotional life to yourself. You learn not to trust others. He described his life as highly compartmentalized. As he attempted to shake off the sadness that overcame him as he shared this with me, he joked wryly that his best friend is a cigarette. The Jamaican and Zimbabwean youth I spoke with were not as bleak in their reflections but still echoed his basic message. It was a struggle to accept that they possessed something of value to offer society.

People Are Going to Know Who I Am

Constituents were reluctant to participate in activities that increased their public visibility. Constituents possessed legitimate fear of violence and social harm (Chapter 1). Their private lives were closely guarded. Developing a "political face" was profoundly challenging because of the degree of personal exposure and risk it required. Akoni said that constituents' deep-seated reluctance to adopt a public profile proved a perennial challenge. Getting constituents' stories and experiences in front of policymakers, health care providers, and other duty bearers is essential to advocacy. But that requires constituents are willing to be seen. Eithan noted his own reluctance to become involved in advocacy stemmed from the concern of public disclosure of his sexual orientation. Reflecting on his first volunteer leadership opportunity, he said:

> I was sent the information that [organization] were looking for applicants. Then [name] who worked here—we used to go to school together—so he sent me the information and said that I should apply. I wasn't sure if I should apply because I was like "No, I don't think I am ready for this. People are going to know who I am and say things." And at the time I was not in the best of places with my family.

Once he overcame this reluctance, he gradually became more involved in civic activities. The path he took initially comprised volunteer opportunities that were not overtly focused on LGBT issues, such as joining with several volunteer groups to clean up an intercoastal waterway.

Concern about adopting a public face was also rooted in fears of professional and personal harm. In Cameroon, advocates complained about the reluctance of older people, by which they meant those in their 30s, 40s, and 50s, to become involved in associations such as Affirmative Action. Engagement posed significant risk to older men's social position. In 2003, the Cameroonian newspaper *The Anecdote* published a list of 50 Cameroonian men suspected of being gay, spoiling their reputations, endangering them and their families, and leading to the murder of an activist named on the list (Brokovitch, 2018). Other papers published similar lists immediately before and after *The Anecdote* (Awondo, 2016). A few months before my first visit to the country, a new list naming 82 people began to circulate on social media. This time, the list included youth, too, imperiling their access to the resources provided to them by their families, such as housing, food, clothing, and school fees, and jeopardizing their safety in a country known for its high rates of violent attacks on adolescent and young adult sexual and gender minority people. Although reluctance on the part of older people to become involved concerned Guy, a Cameroonian activist, he understood its origins, describing the fallout that followed from the lists of names published in the newspapers. The absence of older men in the movement worried him in part due to cultural expectations governing young people's behavior toward adults, and especially authority figures. Older men, he argued, do not face the same danger of violating the cultural norm of deference to elders as do youth. Older men are better positioned to engage in advocacy with policymakers and traditional leaders. While Guy was explaining why he strongly desired to see more older men involved in advocacy, my translator, Chantal, a former youth advocate herself, finished his thought. "In Africa, we say a baby elephant can't defeat an adult elephant," she said. "When you are still small, you have to respect the position of the adult and take the time to grow up." Guy quickly agreed, noting youth may also lack the resources, connections, and savvy to move issues forward. "We are youth," he said, referring to himself and the people willing to volunteer with or work for associations like his. "The movement is youth. And, we have to learn. Learn more. How women have done. How to create collaboration with the National Assembly. How to make a local position. How to discuss with big partners. How to build some ways to carry out our fight."

For some constituents, not knowing where or how to engage was more the issue. Entry points to social change activity and finding networks of peers took time and effort to discover. When I asked Dymond about the participation of other transgender people in political and civic issues, she said that few participate because there are few spaces available to engage. When she described her own journey to Project ACT leadership, Dymond noted that she had long believed she should, and could, do something to improve the lives of her community. "I didn't know how to make that difference or that impact," she explained. Her path was paved once she found J-FLAG.

Like Eithan, once connected to the group, she gradually took on greater responsibility, becoming a representative of transgender people in multiple public and policy influence arenas.

The Project ACT activists reported that few among their constituents were ready to claim their right to health care or access systems of redress because they lacked awareness of the rights they might claim or feared claiming them. On the one hand, activists observed that constituents were unaware of policies to protect them from discrimination, whether those be statements in their national constitution or in national or institutional policies. For instance, Halima remarked that in training constituents in Ghana, she found it was common that men lacked any knowledge of the Ghanaian Patients' Charter,[5] which specifies the right of all Ghanaians to access health care free from discrimination. On the other hand, constituents were reluctant to use existing mechanisms of redress because they believed nothing would be done in response to their complaints. Complaining might also call undesired attention to them. In Jamaica, despite the existence of a national client complaint mechanism for health care and a national diversity policy on how police must respond to and record incidents of violence and harassment, people fail to use these mechanisms out of a combination of learned skepticism, a tendency to minimize the significance of their experiences, and fear of making their situation worse. Akoni explained:

> When you look at the 2016 report that we had published which had surveyed about 316 LGBT people, we found that the data was almost similar to how people felt about other things. People didn't want to make reports to the police for various reasons. And the top reasons for not wanting to report an assault, for example, is that they feel the police would do nothing. Or that they would be further victimized. Or that the incident is too minor to make a report about. And that's something that we see in national data. . . . People just did not believe the police would do anything, if they made a report. And that someone will know that they made a report and [they will] be further victimized.[6]

Preparing Communities for Action

The Project ACT partners took on the tasks of community mobilization and preparation for engaging in advocacy through a combination of strategies to prompt healing and personal insight, educate constituents on the rights they were entitled to claim, and provide constituents safe and nurturing pathways of opportunity. For most of the partners, addressing internalized stigma and assisting constituents to cultivate a sense of self-worth served as their point of departure. The tactics used to create healing ranged from formal workshops to the establishment of ongoing settings for community members to discuss community concerns and challenges. The work of the Sexual Rights Centre in Zimbabwe and J-FLAG in Jamaica reflect these two different approaches.

Addressing Internalized Stigma in Zimbabwe: Looking In, Looking Out

The advocacy tactics that the Sexual Rights Centre adopted as part of Project ACT relied on their constituents to generate strong demand for affirming services, document stigma and discrimination in health care provision, and contribute to training health care workers, as Promise did. The Sexual Rights Centre staff believed that none of this could occur without first remedying internalized stigma (Chapter 1) and fostering a sense of community among gay and bisexual men. The Sexual Rights Centre began its efforts to address internalized stigma by offering 30 community members—mostly late adolescents and young adults—a 3-day workshop designed to foster positive self-regard and interpersonal sensitivity. Members of the Centre's two gay and bisexual male collectives were well-represented among those who participated in the workshop. The Centre selected the *Looking In, Looking Out Identity* workshop (LILO) developed by the Namibian-based organization Positive Vibes (Positive Vibes, nd) as its curriculum. Positive Vibes developed the LILO workshop series for the Eastern and Southern African context; it has been implemented widely in the region. The workshops are grounded in Paulo Freire's principles of liberatory education (Freire, 1970). Consistent with Freire's teaching, the workshops emphasize recovering participants' sense of dignity and humanity and exploring the nature of their oppression. The workshops' design and content mirror that of psychoeducational and empowerment workshops observed to be effective in reducing HIV internalized stigma (see, for example, Ma et al., 2019). They also mirror other psychological frameworks rooted in social justice education and activism. The radical healing framework, for example, emphasizes collectivism, critical consciousness, radical hope, strength, resistance, and cultural authenticity and self-knowledge (French et al., 2020). Individualistic notions of wellness are replaced by connectedness and community, and these are the prerequisites to activism and social change.

The *LILO Identity* workshop addresses the stigma associated with sexual orientation and gender expression. An underlying premise of the workshop is that people must connect structural stigma and discrimination to their individual experiences as a precursor to being able to work in solidarity with and for others. The workshop's activities encourage participants to achieve self-acceptance and a holistic self-view, while simultaneously fostering their critical consciousness about the effects of discrimination and prejudice based on sexual orientation and gender identity and expression. The workshop's exercises highlight and foster appreciation of the diversity among sexual and gender minority people. Building a sense of community and common cause cut through the workshop's activities. The workshop explicitly promotes participants' awareness of concrete actions they can take individually and collectively to undo the interpersonal, community, and structural stigma and discrimination the community endures.

All but one of the young men I met with in Zimbabwe that July had participated in a *LILO Identity* workshop. Everyone who participated characterized the workshop as a life-changing experience. During our small-group conversations, the young men described in vivid detail the key moments in the workshop that they had experienced as revelatory. A visualization exercise in which they were instructed to imagine their future selves came up frequently as especially eye-opening and transformative. Through crafting an imagined potential future, young men recounted that they came to see themselves in "three dimensions," often for the first time. "I realized this is not a career," one recalled, referring to the way in which the exercise enabled him to redefine himself as more than his sexual orientation. "I came to know about myself," another remarked. "I discovered I am someone," a third added.

Several of the young men noted that the *LILO Identity* workshop helped begin to heal deep divides that exist locally between transgender and gay and bisexual people. During my first visit to Zimbabwe, I joined the Sexual Rights Centre staff at their 3-day annual strategic planning retreat. The Centre staff and the leadership of the six collectives were all present. During the retreat, I sat between the head of the transgender collective, Aneni, and the head of the male sex worker collective, Dumi, so I could talk to them both. Throughout the retreat, at times finding the common denominator across the diverse communities that the collectives represented proved a struggle, but that struggle was most pronounced for Aneni and the transgender collective she represented. On the first day of the retreat, the morning activities included taking stock of successes and failures from the prior year. Inadequate attention to transgender people and "forcing trans people into the MSM/HIV box" emerged as an item on the list of things that had gone poorly. But 2 days later, when Aneni presented on the needs of her collective, a heated and tense discussion arose at her suggestion that safer spaces for transgender people could and should be established within the Centre. She suddenly found herself under attack. Aneni vigorously defended her position, but she eventually shrank into her chair. Penya, in her even-handed, soothing, and Socratic leadership style, urged her staff to consider the shared experiences and concerns among those around the table.

The day after the retreat, Mbuso affirmed my observations that an undercurrent of tension was present between the transgender and gay and bisexual cisgender male constituencies. When I asked him whether he thought that the Centre was gender affirming in general, I wrongly assumed that in framing his response he might comment on the cisgender female staff, the Centre's long-standing advocacy on the rights of female sex workers, or the collective representing lesbian and bisexual women. Instead, his initial response to my question was that he did not want to comment. Then he explained that he did not understand much about transgender people. He characterized the divide between cisgender gay and bisexual men and transgender women as a barrier for the Centre. "We don't understand each other," he said. He reflected on the history of interaction between the two communities. When transgender people initially pursued an alliance with the local gay male community and Penya warmly welcomed their involvement in the Centre, Mbuso said the response from gay and bisexual men was " 'No, we don't associate with you guys. We are different.'" He paused. "But at the end of the day, the things they are affected by, they are the ones that affect us." He concluded our conversation on gender by stating that the gay and bisexual male community were novices when it came to working in solidarity with transgender people but were finally starting to learn.

The young men who attended the *LILO Identity* workshop believed they gained novel insight on transgender experiences in the workshop. They came to appreciate the differences among sexual orientation, sexual identity, gender identity, and gender expression. The workshop helped them to value the diverse community to which they belong. We are not "a hive mind," as one put it. This young man spoke in detail about how the workshop assisted him to achieve what scholars refer to as positive marginality (e.g., Dutt and Grabe, 2014; Mayo, 1982). In the workshop, he discovered the privileges that his bisexuality conferred on him. He identified ways he could use his privilege to help others, especially transgender people. Others echoed his perception that they felt better prepared to help cisgender and transgender community members and to act with greater self-awareness in how they treated others. One shared a story of a cathartic moment after the *LILO Identity* workshop in which he helped a cisgender man better understand transgender issues. He was in a semipublic setting and overheard a man make loud misstatements about a transgender person who happened to be in the man's earshot. He intervened. He used the quadrant model he had learned in the training, which distinguished sex from gender identity, to address the man's misstatements.[7] "In that moment, I could be a representative for transgender people. I could prevent a verbal attack," he shared, attributing his ability to do so to his *LILO Identity* training.

As they spoke about their experience, the young men made multiple mentions of developing a sense of unity and perceiving those they had met through the workshop as a loving family. Young men observed the workshop fostered a sense of community among them, diminishing social isolation, and increasing their exposure to each other and to peer role models. Young men claimed the workshop enabled them to become models of self-pride. It offered them "armor against homophobia." The young men offered me only two criticisms of the *LILO Identity* workshop: they wanted it to last longer and for more workshops to be made available to members of the local community who had not had the opportunity to participate.

Addressing Internalized Stigma in Jamaica: Community Conversations

The Jamaican approach to addressing internalized stigma was decidedly less formal than the approach adopted by the Sexual Rights Centre (and partners in countries such as Ghana) that chose to rely on a curriculum-driven workshop informed by popular education principles. Yet the Jamaican approach proved no less influential in prompting the introspection and consciousness raising that precedes successful community mobilization and can foster citizen engagement in public-facing advocacy. J-FLAG pursued its traditional efforts to pursue policy change, raise the visibility of LGBT concerns in the national media, and build constructive bridges to the business, policing, criminal justice, education, health care, social service, and government sectors to improve the national climate for LGBT people. J-FLAG also focused its efforts on fostering a nascent transgender policy agenda and building the capacity of a fledgling transgender organization named TransWave[8] to break down the barriers to access to HIV care for transgender women.

J-FLAG's approach to addressing the impacts of stigma on constituents' self-perceptions was driven in no small part by the formative nature of the Jamaican transgender movement. Dymond, who spearheaded this part of Project ACT, often commented to me that for all intents and purposes, transgender people "did not exist" and are "invisible" in Jamaica. They are not in the public eye. They are not part of national health surveillance efforts. Transgender people, she observed, barely see themselves as part of a community of people with a set of common concerns. In one conversation, Dymond pointed to an attitudinal survey of the public conducted about 3 years before the start of Project ACT as evidence of how absent transgender people were from the national scene. She noted that every question posed about transgender people was typically responded to with "Don't know." "There is not a lot of information already related to trans people in Jamaica," she explained. "Lots about LGB people, but not a lot about trans people." As she spoke about the lack of awareness of transgender people in Jamaica, I recalled J-FLAG's 20th anniversary fete, which was held at one of the only hotels in Kingston willing to host J-FLAG's events.[9] As I was departing, a taxi arrived conveying several transgender women on their way to the gathering. As the women exited the car and headed to the entrance, their cabdriver half-stood through the driver's side window of his cab, as if paralyzed. His left arm dangled on the exterior of the car door, his head and chest protruding through the open window, his eyes wide and mouth agape as he gawked at the women walking away, oblivious to the impatient drivers queued up behind him. Although he appeared cartoonish as he stood out the cab's window, his puzzlement and disbelief were plain. As a woman traveling alone throughout Project ACT, my safety was always uppermost in my mind. It informed my choices of where to stay, what to wear, how to get around, and where I should not go alone. Watching his expression as the three women walked past me, I could not help myself from worrying whether they would safely make it home that evening.

A second reason driving the informality of the Jamaican approach concerned the need to create a community-driven safe space that might help overcome the anxieties and fears transgender community members harbored about the extent of their welcome. Among Dymond's first efforts when she began at J-FLAG was drafting its current organizational policy to ensure the organization is safe and affirming. Finally, the approach J-FLAG pursued suited its organizational culture, which balances the grueling demands of sophisticated policy analysis and national government advocacy, with opportunities for casual social time imbued with playfulness.

J-FLAG launched a series of facilitated community conversations that were open to the J-FLAG community. Each of the conversations focused on a community-generated topic concerning internalized stigma, stigmatizing dynamics within the community, sexual health and well-being, or human rights issues. Conversations were facilitated by someone knowledgeable of the nominated topic, whether a staff member from J-FLAG or TransWave, a community member, or a representative of an allied organization. The J-FLAG approach had the advantage of allowing responsiveness to salient dynamics and contemporary events. Among the earliest conversations were two sessions that resonated deeply with the community, one focused on body image, body shaming, and body positivity and the second on colorism within the community. According to Dymond, the body image discussion "brought out so much that people actually broke down in tears." A transgender youth I interviewed described the conversation as "powerful" because she loves doing drag but is often told she is not pretty enough. Recounting what she learned through the conversation, she said, "There is no one definition of what is a woman. It was uplifting."

A catalytic discussion on colorism arose in reaction to the controversy that ensued when the popular hip-hop and dancehall artist, Spice, released a video in which she had whitened her skin. Candice explained:

> We've kind of framed it on the terms of what is happening within society now, and how that might impact you as an individual, particularly as an LGBT individual. What had happened prior is a very popular dancehall artist, Spice, put out a music video, where . . . you are familiar, with blackface?
>
> *Robin: Mm-hmm.*
>
> Yeah. What she had done was done makeup so that she was significantly lighter than she was. We kind of had a conversation about if anyone else had done this, would the reaction have been different? Because she, Spice, is controversial in that sense. And she is well loved and liked by Jamaicans. But, if someone else had done this, would it have been received differently and how is that perceived on our own ideas of self? Bleaching is a very popular thing in Jamaica. How do we perceive that as individuals and the associations with lighter-skinned persons as opposed to darker-skinned persons and the privileges those persons can enjoy?

Dymond cited this conversation as significant for also raising the tensions between LGB people and transgender people and the extent to which intersectional stigmas are perpetuated within the community itself:

> LBG people having a problem with trans people but also looking at skin color and how the color of their skin and how that type of colorism or mindset fits into the conversation of self-stigma. . . . They appreciated the conversation because it's things that they never thought about before. And they never realized that they themselves are perpetrators of certain things and how those things can be barriers to them in achieving what they need to achieve—specifically as it relates to their

health. For a lot of them they are afraid to go to these places because they think they won't be able to blend in and they'll stick out or someone might out them or they won't be treated fairly. Not just because they are LBGT, but also because they are LBGT and poor or because they are LGBT and dark.

Those I interviewed often referred to this conversation as the first of several that caused them to pause and reflect on interpersonal insensitivities and biases perpetuated within their community. Dymond noted that, through word of mouth, demand for more conversations increased quickly after the first few gatherings. People began to bring friends. As the conversations evolved, topics included coming out, mental health, health care, healthy relationships, dealing with the police, and responding to violence.

On my second visit to Jamaica, I interviewed several young transgender women who had participated in community conversations. Although each woman offered criticisms of the groups, each also emphasized the conversations were personally meaningful. They came away with the clear message that they could and should be their authentic selves without apology. In addition to the many useful things that they learned about navigating in society and claiming their rights, the conversations left them feeling better about themselves and less alone. Their criticisms of the groups were wide ranging, including the topics chosen, the heavy tilt toward the concerns of middle-class participants, and scheduling, but each woman would take every opportunity to attend future conversations, and each would continue to encourage her friends to join in them. Just as in Zimbabwe, these convenings permitted constituents to explore their shared experiences of vulnerability, reduced their sense of social isolation, increased their belief in their self-worth, and led to the establishment of new or stronger connections to others with whom they could identify.

When Claiming Rights Goes Wrong

For a small number of constituents, the outcomes of their newfound sense of self-worth and awareness of the rights they should claim did not always lead to desired consequences, at least in the short term. Although rare, in a few cases when a constituent claimed a right or expressed their identity proudly and publicly, it led to trouble that required partners to intervene. The Project ACT partners were prepared to act in these cases, having developed response and support systems for constituents over the course of their organizations' existence. Even so, two incidents, one from Ghana and another from Jamaica, point to the importance of organizational preparedness for similar occurrences.

In Ghana and other project countries, extortion is a widespread problem for gay, bisexual, and other men who have sex with men. Our Ghanaian partner's internalized stigma reduction workshop addressed the rights its participants might claim, including freedom from extortion. Participants learned to report incidents of stigma and discrimination, including extortion attempts, to our partner, which many did.

But several sought to handle an instance of blackmail on their own. In one case, a man reported his landlord's son to the police without engaging our partner first, as the workshop trainer had counseled. Halima explains:

> And then, there was another case of a guy being harassed in his apartment by the landlord's son and a friend. They went into his room, picked up his stuff, and took them away. And he went straight to report to the police because he said we told him that if anything happens, he should go straight to the police station and report the case first. So, he reported to the police before even calling us. And, when he reported another time, the guys [who stole his belongings] went back to report him. And *he* got arrested [based on the blackmailers' assertions] that he was actually MSM. Then they [the police] demanded for bail money for him to get out. So, he paid the bail money. Meanwhile he wasn't supposed to do that. But lucky for him, he reported them the first time.

Our partner used the prior police reports and recordings of telephone interactions the man had made with his blackmailers to persuade the police commander that the man should not have been arrested or bail demanded of him. The commander returned his bail money and ensured the blackmailers returned the money, phone, and other belongings they had stolen from his lodging.

In Jamaica, a transgender woman who was a few weeks shy of the age of 18 and who still lived with her parents agreed to participate in a Pride photoshoot, buoyed by a sense of elation and desire to live authentically that was fostered by the community conversations. Under most circumstances, such as at school, she presented herself as male. The photos ended up on social media, where they were quickly discovered by someone who knew her family. The images then rapidly circulated in her neighborhood and to her parents. Threats to her safety followed, prompting her to leave home immediately, despite complete material dependence on her family. I spoke with her 1 month after she had sought temporary safe shelter. Tears formed at the edge of her eyes as she spoke about how desperately she missed her mother, grandmother, and sister. She ached to see them. She no longer had any idea how she would be able to pay to complete her schooling. But she took great comfort that she had joined a united family through her participation in the community conversations and at the opportunities those conversations had opened to her. "I know I have the right to be heard," she said. The incident gave her the strength not to care what others think. "I learned about pride and that it is a celebration of my freedom." Finding her community and developing her sense of agency made the separation from her natal family bearable.

Providing Advocacy Opportunities

Empowerment requires participation. Project ACT partners created diverse roles for their constituents that were essential to carrying out local advocacy and which simultaneously created pathways for constituents' empowerment. Across Project ACT countries, constituents were called upon to collect evidence of stigma and discrimination in health care provision using variations on mystery patient methodology; to assume a diversity of peer leadership roles; and to engage in sharing their experiences of stigma in trainings, on social media, and in other venues. These advocacy tasks allow activists to raise awareness of stigma and discrimination and make abstract concepts such as stigma into concrete human-interest stories (Mitchell et al., 2022). Mystery patient methods typically involve deploying mock clients to document quality of service provision and policy conformity. Although each of these opportunities differs in its demands and risks, the systems of training, mentorship, and support developed by local partners enabled constituents to succeed in and sustain their participation in these roles. Constituents took to these roles most eagerly and successfully in the countries in which the Project ACT partners provided ample social, material, and psychological support.

Documenting Stigma and Discrimination in Health Care

In Cameroon, Ghana, and Zimbabwe, Project ACT partners relied on constituents to document stigma and discrimination.[10] Several implemented innovations inspired by mystery patient methodology (see, for example, Baptiste et al., 2020; Chin-Quee et al., 2006; Collins et al., 2017; Daouk-Oyry et al., 2018; Liambila et al., 2010; McGinn et al., 2019) to collect systematic data on discrimination in the provision of health care. Approaches were tailored in ways that the partners believed were best suited to their context.[11] The data collected by mystery patients were used to persuade area health care personnel to redress stigma and discrimination, guide the development and implementation of redress and improvement plans, and identify facilities whose providers and practices were experienced positively.

Peer Mobilization and Leadership Development

Peer mobilization was central to the activities in Zimbabwe. Among the 30 participants in the Zimbabwe *LILO Identity* workshops, 10 men were invited to engage in additional training and eventually to take on the leadership role of a peer mobilizer. As peer mobilizers, young men were tasked with generating demand for, and linking their peers to, health care; ensuring peers documented their health care interactions using a community-designed stigma checklist; accompanying peers to health care visits to offer support; and, if needed, acting as patient advocates. The peer mobilizers represented local gay and bisexual men on an ad hoc committee, along with Centre staff and health care personnel from area facilities. The committee met on a quarterly basis to review and discuss patient experiences of stigma and discrimination captured in the completed checklists and to develop redress plans. The peer mobilizers engaged in policy advocacy meetings with politicians and other duty bearers and designed their own community advocacy actions.

The 10 young men received specialized training in preparation for taking on their charge. The *LILO Voice* (Positive Vibes, no date) workshop formed the foundation of their additional training. The *LILO Voice* workshop prepares its participants for advocacy work through activities that closely examine how power and privilege operate and the role of predominant narratives and counternarratives in shaping, maintaining, and challenging oppression. The peer mobilizers also received specialized training in mystery patient methods, counseling skills, HIV, and sexual health. The 10 men received ongoing mentoring and coaching from seasoned Centre staff, principally Mbuso, Mandla, and Thandi. Reflecting on their role, the mobilizers noted they provided the foundation for the advocacy work and brought the Sexual Rights Centre closer to the community. Peer mobilization "forced them to be solution givers."

In Burundi, Cameroon, Jamaica, Côte d'Ivoire, and Zimbabwe, mobilization and leadership development occurred among small community-led organizations, several of which were not yet registered with their governments or in a position to be direct recipients of donor funding. The partners invested in developing the capacity of these smaller community-led organizations through training and inviting their participation in project activities. They also engaged in professional development and mentoring of organizational leaders. In Zimbabwe, for instance, organizational leadership development occurred principally through engagement of two collectives in nearly all aspects of the work of the project. In Jamaica, at the outset of Project ACT, TransWave employed only one person: Dymond. Leadership development focused principally on her professional development in policy advocacy (e.g., developing policy briefs and shadow reports), expanding opportunities to link her to regional, national, and international networks and activities, and supporting her ability to mentor other community members. It also included coaching on activities, such as organizing a day-long national transgender health conference. MPact staff contributed to these efforts, providing supplementary training, on-site assistance, and linkages to resources and opportunities.

Public Engagement and Testimonial

Partners created mechanisms to engage in public speaking and testimonials, letter writing to newspapers, and meetings with duty bearers. These opportunities extended the organizational leadership development work. In Jamaica, constituents composed letters to the editor, participated in small media videos, and spoke on panels. In Cameroon, mystery patients provided testimony of their experience, just as the young people in Zimbabwe did. Constituents in Zimbabwe were mentored through the process of writing about their work and submitting presentation abstracts to national and regional conferences. In Côte d'Ivoire, constituents offered short video testimonials of stigma and discrimination for distribution on social media.

Conclusion

Empowerment theories underscore the importance of learning to see connections between the individual- and community-level suffering that oppressive structures produce (Freiere, 1970). The process by which people achieve this conscientization often
requires engaging with others in forums that heighten their interpersonal sensitivity
and prompt their critical analysis and reflection (Staub & Vollhardt, 2008; Vollhardt,
2009; Vollhardt & Staub, 2011). The LILO Identity workshop and the Community
Conversations helped participants see the ways in which their experiences mirrored
one another's and recognize how they were driven by a complex set of oppressive societal dynamics, dynamics they could mobilize to resist. Finding one another in these
settings created the sense of community that had so long been impeded by the effects
of structural stigma. The LILO curriculum and the informal conversations broke
through constituents' isolation, providing them with the sense of "we" that is essential
to well-being.

Increasing a sense of self-worth and opportunities for meaningful engagement are
critical to national, regional, and global advocacy movements. That is because advocacy, at its core, requires the ability to disrupt and to reveal power structures that sub-
jugate. But to accomplish this, sexual and gender minority people must feel safe and
that they matter to themselves and to others. They must claim their agency in community with others who share lived experiences of oppression. They must be sensitized
to see stigma, discrimination, and structural violence in real time and confidently and
vehemently object to it. This work at the individual level is akin to waking a sleeping
giant. Global movements begin with the essential work of overcoming the traumas
inflicted by homophobia and transphobia, including self-hatred and self-doubt,
and addressing the ways in which these obstruct a sense of belonging (Chapter 1;
Lattanner & Hatzenbuehler, 2023) and of mattering (Prilleltensky & Prilleltensky,
2021). For sexual and gender minority people, the realization that their experiences
of stigma, discrimination, and violence are shared can solidify supportive bonds with
one another. These bonds can extend beyond the local. Community can be realized
beyond the borders of a village or town and reside in global movements. Within these
bonds, promise rises.

6
We Need Allies

It took Chantal several tries before she identified a taxi driver willing to drive us the 7-kilometer distance from Centre Ville to Biyem Assi. I stood on the side of Boulevard du 20 Mai, watching as she flagged down the rare empty cab in search of a driver who would accept the fare she offered and agree not to stop along the way to pick up other passengers, as is the local custom in Cameroon. When she finally hailed me over, we rapidly slid into the sagging backseat before our driver could change his mind. Springs pressed through deep indentations created by the bottoms of countless other passengers. Shifting left or right in search of better cushioning was impossible. My rear inevitably slipped back into the bowl-shaped depression in the worn vinyl seat as our cab sped away from the curb, lurching into the thick of Yaoundé's midday traffic.

We passed the parade viewing stands and then forced our way into a traffic circle choked with cars belching diesel, each driver for themselves. "In Cameroon, we fight with our cars," Chantal quipped, glancing up from the cracked screen of her cellphone, as our driver fearlessly nosed his taxi into every small opening he could. He wedged his cab tightly between two dented vehicles crowding the circle, leaving barely a hand-width of space between our doors and theirs. We crept around, battling our way, until a less obstructed path appeared up a winding slope. We headed southeast through a maze of streets that turned abruptly from pavement to red clay and to pavement again. Eventually, we chugged slowly up a hillside street lined on the left with roadside stalls alongside a masonry retaining wall, and on the right by low-lying buildings constructed into the hill's slope. As we neared the hill's peak, Chantal leaned toward the driver. "Arretez ici, s'il vous plait." (Stop here, please.) We stopped in front of a small storefront. I slid out of the cab, while Chantal stood in the dusty street, unfolding a fistful of francs pulled from the depths of her designer handbag. I followed Chantal as she made her way gingerly uphill on the spiked heels that are her shoe of choice. We proceeded down a steep stone staircase in a narrow alley formed by two closely set buildings. When we reached the bottom, we entered an unmarked door leading us into a small, dimly lit room on the building's lowest level. Chantal and I had come to check on the progress of Project ACT with the staff of a mainstream Cameroonian civil society human rights advocacy organization named Positive Generation, a critical local ally to Project ACT. This chapter describes how the Project ACT partners engaged with allies from diverse societal sectors and involved them in advocacy to address local barriers to care. We characterize the motivations for allyship and the role that allies play in making advocacy possible. We illustrate collaboration

Breaking Barriers. Robin Lin Miller and George Ayala, Oxford University Press. © Oxford University Press 2024.
DOI: 10.1093/oso/9780197647684.003.0007

and allyship as fundamental to advocacy practice. We highlight allyship experiences and obstacles to collaboration from Cote d'Ivoire, Cameroon, and Zimbabwe.

Mainstream Alliances

Advocacy movements benefit from allies, both allies from movements with identical (or nearly identical) concerns and those from movements focused on different social issues but with overlapping root causes (Chapter 2; Mitchell et al., 2022; Rucht, 2004). Allies strengthen partners' efforts, and for many, reciprocally so. Some allies are well positioned to influence duty bearers who play a role in maintaining the local status quo. Some allies possess critical capacities and can bring needed resources to bear. Some provide entry into social, financial, and institutional networks that would otherwise be inaccessible.

Almost every Project ACT partner needed the cooperation and engagement of other community-led organizations to pursue the advocacy they envisioned. These relationships were the fount of mystery patients, of testimonials, of individuals mobilized to claim rights in targeted settings, and of shared intelligence. Little advocacy could occur without their engagement. But the Project ACT partners also needed to leverage allies from outside these familiar cooperating networks. These partnerships did not evolve through happenstance. Instead, they were deliberate, strategic choices to build power at the community, country, and international levels. This often meant collaborating with organizations from the mainstream. Positive Generation was one such ally.

Positive Generation

Among the accomplishments of which Guy, Emil, and Richard are most proud is convincing Positive Generation to collaborate with Affirmative Action and its local network of "identity associations"—the term they use to refer to member-based clubs that we term "community-led organizations." In a country that criminalizes homosexuality and in which homophobic attitudes prevail, convincing a mainstream organization like Positive Generation to work in partnership with Affirmative Action was no small feat. The heart of the advocacy work that occurred in Cameroon depended entirely on the success of this novel alliance. Through this partnership, Affirmative Action and Positive Generation co-designed and implemented a system for measuring stigma and discrimination in high-volume HIV care facilities, trained LGBT community members from nine community-led organizations to assume the role of mystery patients, and developed strategies for sharing data with and providing sensitization to health care providers, government officials, and other duty bearers.

Founded in 1998, Positive Generation began as a movement of university students to promote safer sexual practices and provide HIV information to Cameroon's young people. The group quickly extended its focus to the human rights issues facing people living with HIV and HIV stigma reduction. Holding the Cameroonian government to account to provide adequate health care to people living with HIV became central to the organization's mission. The organization perfected a national treatment access monitoring initiative to collect real-time data on disruptions in access to antiretroviral treatment. According to the Positive Generation staff, their system focuses on accountability to patients' rights: whether treatment ends up being given to patients when they go to health care facilities that are subcontracted to provide it, whether services are charged at the designated government rate, whether providers try to extract fees for what should be a free service, and whether basic elements of HIV services such as HIV pretest and posttest counseling are denied or omitted. Positive Generation uses the data it collects to apply pressure to health care officials to improve the national systems of HIV care and minimize medication supply chain disruptions. The organization's achievements are locally well known and earned it a 2012 designation as the best advocacy program in Africa from One Africa, an honor in which the staff takes immense pride.

The watchdog system that helped Positive Generation earn international praise runs on ongoing, covert surveillance of government health care providers in 62 health districts and over 80 facilities. Using a well-designed sampling strategy and structured observational protocol, a cadre of veteran monitors collect data by making health care visits. Data are analyzed and reported weekly to track trends and to intervene on specific real-time problems in access to treatment. For example, the organization once identified that antiretroviral therapy was unavailable at a primary designated treatment site in the southern region of the country. Upon investigation, Positive Generation uncovered that the director of this facility would not authorize staff to pick up the medication at the regional distribution site because transportation there and back was not a reimbursable expense. Positive Generation intervened, first with the director and then at the divisional level, to ensure the 2-week drought of medication came to an immediate end. Although hard tactics are a last-resort strategy, the organization employs them when necessary to call attention to system failures and a lack of response to their less aggressive strategies. The organization once ceremoniously awarded "poor practices" certificates to each of the facilities with the worst performance among facilities in several regions, publicly shaming these facilities into improving.

Affirmative Action pursued an alliance to leverage Positive Generation's experience and expertise in data collection. At the time, limited data were available to demonstrate the frequency and severity of stigma and discrimination impeding gay and bisexual men's and transgender women's access to HIV care.[1] Affirmative Action staff and board members believed evidence was key to successful advocacy for improving access. Collecting watchdog data was a new tactic for the Affirmative Action staff. None of them possessed the expertise in the sampling, measurement, data collection, or statistics that are fundamental to this type of surveillance. The Affirmative Action staff viewed obtaining these data as groundbreaking for their organization's maturing capacity in advocacy and for national efforts to break down barriers due to stigma and discrimination. Gaston reflected the view, shared among his colleagues, that lacking solid data was an impediment to Affirmative Action's advocacy:

> When we do not have data, it is difficult to implement activities or run activities that yield a result. Meanwhile, by having all this information, we'll be able to see if the problem is coming from health practitioners or if the problem is not even at the level of the beneficiaries. So, it will be very important. And this is a really ground-breaking and innovative project.

It was a groundbreaking effort for Positive Generation, too. To the best of their staff's knowledge, data that track routine acts of stigma and discrimination in health care interactions for any of Cameroon's most vulnerable populations did not exist. Data specific to gay men and transgender women were rarely collected, and certainly not part of any ongoing national surveillance protocols of which they were aware. The last data they had seen on the stigmatization experiences of gay men were some 16 years old. Positive Generation could pioneer an entirely novel effort through this collaboration. According to Gaston, the partnership also facilitated Affirmative Action's first direct advocacy engagement with health care facilities. Positive Generation routinely put pressure on these systems, something Affirmative Action desired to do. For Guy, the alliance represented a first, not simply for the data it could produce and the ways in which it would change the nature of Affirmative Action's relationship to local health care facilities. For him, working with an ally that was not from the LBGT sector and was a long-standing mainstream player in the HIV advocacy movement in Cameroon demonstrated Affirmative Action's credibility. "It is good to work with Positive Generation as an ally because they are not an LGBTI organization," he observed. "We need to expand our allies. To show we can carry big programs. To show we are credible." The legitimacy conferred on Affirmative Action through an allegiance with Positive Generation was valuable currency. The relationship between these two collaborators highlights the reciprocal benefits of allyships between mainstream and community-led organizations.

REPMASCI

Another vital alliance with a prominent mainstream organization drove the advocacy work in Côte d'Ivoire. Alternative Côte d'Ivoire extended an existing alliance with Réseau des professionnels des médias, des arts et des sports engagés dans la lutte contre le Sida et les autres pandémies (Network of media, arts and sports professionals engaged in the fight against AIDS and other pandemics) (REPMASCI) to build on the lessons the organizations had learned through a trial partnership that preceded the start of Project ACT. REPMASCI's mission is to ensure accurate reporting on epidemics that endanger the health of Ivoirians and to increase national reporting on

HIV. To fulfill its mission, the organization provides capacity building and education for journalists. It sponsors awards for excellence in HIV reporting, among other endeavors. REPMASCI is deeply enmeshed with and supported by the national AIDS control program of the Ministère de la Santè et de l'Hygiène Publique. The organization has a broad reach into national networks for journalists. It is a partner to several unions, including the Union Nationale of Journalistes of Côte d'Ivoire and the Union of Radios in Proximity Côte d'Ivoire. Its links to these networks and its government backing positions REPAMSCI as a key national influencer on health and HIV reportage. For groups such as Alternative Côte d'Ivoire, the relationship to REPMASCI had opened doors through which the organization might shift the predominate anti-LGBT narratives in media. Project ACT permitted Alternative Côte d'Ivoire to keep its foot in that door.

The original partnership between the two organizations developed under an initiative of Institut Panos Afrique de L'Ouest. Institut Panos Afrique de L'Ouest is an independent, locally led member of an international network of similar institutes. The Panos Institutes originated in the Global North to advance the use of reliable, fact-based information in the public sphere to promote debate, pluralism, and democracy in the Global South. For Institut Panos Afrique de L'Ouest, addressing violations of LGBT rights is a priority under its human rights program. Institut Panos Afrique de L'Ouest's mission includes encouraging the production of balanced information in media about LGBT people and their concerns, increased coverage of rights violations perpetrated against LBGT people, and the inclusion of LGBT people in all forms of media. A 3-year initiative to pursue these objectives in Senegal, Cameroon, and Côte d'Ivoire brought REMPASCI and Alternative Côte d'Ivoire together. In their initial alliance, the two groups trained Ivoirian journalists on LGBT human rights to encourage them to report on stories that sat at the intersection of HIV and sexual and gender minority rights.

Although REPMASCI, Alternative Côte d'Ivoire, and the Institut Panos Afrique de L'Ouest considered the initial project an overall success, REPMASCI and Alternative Côte d'Ivoire learned hard lessons through their first 3 years of collaboration. Recruiting journalists who were willing to be trained to report on LGBT concerns proved difficult. Among those who were trained, many declined to go on to report on the issues. Only a small cadre of 14 journalists proved themselves willing to do the kind of reporting that REMPASCI and Alternative Côte d'Ivoire envisioned. In the Panos project, those journalists encountered unanticipated obstacles. The managing editors and radio station managers who make the decisions about what pieces will run or be heard on air demurred, passing up on their stories. LGBT community members also proved reluctant to interact with journalists because the visibility that resulted from engaging with the media increased their vulnerability to violence and discrimination. Under Project ACT, REPMASCI and Alternative Côte d'Ivoire committed to extend their alliance. They trained managing editors and station managers and tried to expand the core of trained journalists. They brought trained journalists and LGBT community-led organizations together to prepare the community-led organizations to work with journalists. Community-led organizations also received training in the creation of videos appropriate to disseminate on small media platforms. The community-created videos documented experiences of stigma and discrimination and showed how stigma infringed on the right to health and well-being.

Facilitators and Challenges to Allyships

Although the collaborations established by Affirmative Action and Alternative Côte D'Ivoire were essential to the project and succeeded in many respects, neither of them was problem-free. The nature of the challenges differed. For the alliance between Positive Generation and Affirmative Action, adapting the Positive Generation methodology to account for the risks to LGBT mystery patients' personal safety in Cameroon's hostile context presented a steeper learning curve than either collaborator anticipated. For Positive Generation, an organization accustomed to working with seasoned mystery patients, deploying a cadre of people for whom this was their first experience of data collection required more intensive supervision and support than they were accustomed to providing. Simultaneously, Positive Generation had to cope with a project budget so modest that its typical 5-day training for new mystery patients had to be collapsed to a mere 2 days. As we describe in greater detail in Chapter 7, it took time for the two partners to figure out how to adapt Positive Generation's standard approach to suit the circumstances and to engage the nine community-led identity organizations that were supplying the mystery patients meaningfully in that redesign process. The two groups also struggled over ownership of the data and reports. Positive Generation's stance on their methodology and reports is proprietary. The two organizations had not developed a common view of who was partnering with whom and what it meant for Affirmative Action to be in the lead. At one point during the project, Affirmative Action was challenged to obtain summaries of the data being collected through the mystery patient activity. "We had to exert pressure and bypass Positive Generation to get the reports. We went directly to the CBOs." These challenges underscore the value of establishing a clear and detailed Memorandum of Understanding between partners in advance, including the bases for resolutions of disputes and ownership of processes and products.

The common interest of both Positive Generation and Affirmative Action to a rights-based approach to addressing HIV and to evidence-informed advocacy permitted them to navigate through the challenges they encountered successfully. The like-minded nature of the mission of the two entities and their similar leadership and managerial styles proved essential to their ability to adjust to the nature of what they encountered in the field together. Both organizations are strategic and planful in their activities. Both are well managed and led by leaders whom the staff and others outside the organizations deeply respect. Each possesses staff that enjoy and are committed to their work. Staff seldom turn over.

More significant tensions existed between REPMASCI and Alternative Côte d'Ivoire, tensions that were never fully resolved. The tensions between these two allies emanated in part from the vastly different operating cultures of the two organizations, especially their starkly different communication and leadership styles. Despite REMPASCI's strength of commitment to better journalism about LGBT people, the differences in how these partners functioned and in their expectations of one another caused for an uneasy alliance. In the interviews I conducted on three separate visits, no one ever spoke in a positive manner about the way in which Alternative Côte d'Ivoire was managed or of its leader's manner of interacting principally through intermediaries. People routinely pointed out that he was never present at meetings, which irked them. Among the more striking features of my three weeklong visits to Côte d'Ivoire was that I never saw or met him, despite spending part of nearly every day at the office. He did not attend the Cambodia kickoff retreat, one of only two executive leaders who were absent. He was not present at either of two audiences I held with the director of Côte d'Ivoire's Programme National de Lutte Contre le Sida and his senior staff. In the second of these meetings, another evaluator was present. She worked for a French government agency who also happened to be site visiting the organization during the same week. By the point of that meeting, I assumed the leader had no particular interest in me or in my ambassadorial role for MPact. (I had plenty of indication he was in town from his staff.) I later learned he made no effort to meet with the MPact country lead when he visited, which the country lead also found peculiar. I was told by interviewees they seldom, if ever, interacted with him. Instead, he conveyed precise instructions on what they must do via staff like Claude, who often had to serve as his mouthpiece. Interviewees complained of orders to show up for meetings at the last minute. They characterized this style of interaction and communication as highly disrespectful. His staff, too, were subject to commands at all hours of night and day. At times, these had nothing to do with their work function. These just-in-time demands forced staff to make last-minute changes to their work and personal plans. They lived with it, but unhappily. The MPact country lead observed that the only way Project ACT could have succeeded resulted from how hard-working Claude was. The country lead said he was also struck by how seldom the staff appeared to find joy in their work. Their deep commitment to the issues and to sexual and gender minority rights did not appear to translate to commitment to and love of the organization.

Major disputes about project finances also soured the partnership. Through to the project's conclusion, REPMASCI and the journalists bitterly insisted that the financial and material resources promised to them remained unfulfilled. At each site visit, REPMASCI's representatives and journalists complained that equipment pledged to them to enable their reporting had not materialized. REPMASCI had not received half of its promised compensation. Interviewees would often stop mid-sentence and point at my $80 Olympus audio recorder, which was positioned between us; they were to have received one just like it to enable them to conduct interviews. Funds for recorders were a line item in the budget, but only a handful of recorders were handed out at an end-of-project party as prizes. "This project suffered from financial corruption," one journalist claimed. "We did not get the materials or funds to support the work." Alternative's staff countered these claims by asserting that the journalists' expectations had been "spoiled" by luxurious meetings at beach resort hotels during the PANOS-funded project. Project ACT, they said, was comparatively under-resourced and understaffed. Only two of the four funded staff on the project contributed effort to it, they said. In the end, the partners never found a way to address their ongoing dissatisfaction with one another's ways of operating. The partnership between these allies, though it proceeded, was chronically strained by questions of Alternative Côte d'Ivoire's financial trustworthiness and management style. As noted by Mitchell and colleagues (2022), willingness to share power and resources and to view oneself as others do are vital aspects of leading successful alliances. Alternative Côte d'Ivoire struggled in these aspects of successful collaboration. At the same time, institutional allies of LGBT community-led organizations must challenge the traditional power dynamics within their own relationships to these groups in order for these partnerships to succeed (Russell & Bohan, 2016). In both the case of Positive Generation and REPMASCI, the fact that LGBT-identity organizations held the purse strings and were in the lead was, in and of itself, a challenge to the status quo. That may not have always sat comfortably.

Lady's Cooperation Association Sportive

In the advocacy literature, allies are defined as nonmembers of the societal group that the advocacy initiative is expressly intended to benefit. As people who are assumed not to share the oppressed or stigmatized status that gives rise to the need for an advocacy initiative, allies may possess social power and privilege that can prove helpful. Inherent in this conceptualization of an ally is the notion of championing *someone else's* cause and leveraging one's own social power on the behalf of that someone. REPMASCI and its staff, the journalists who REPMASCI trained, the staff of Positive Generation, and many other groups and individuals who contributed to Project ACT fit this conventional definition of an ally. Staff who worked at MPact and at several of the partnering organizations, such as Affirmative Action and the Sexual Rights Centre, fit this definition, too. As Richard explained to me, having straight people working under the leadership of gay people at Affirmative Action was a huge source of strength because others would see "heterosexuals battling for the rights of the community." But the notion of an ally as someone who is completely outside the experience of the societal group whose cause is championed does not apply equally to all of Project ACT's allies. Some allies possessed an identity that positioned them at a point of social intersection and interconnected experience with the gay and bisexual men and transgender women who were the focus of the project. The members of an association in Yaoundé founded to address gender-based violence illustrate this intersectionality.

Roughly 5 years before Affirmative Action became a legal entity, a group of professional female athletes founded an association to combat the flagrant abuses experienced by players on Cameroon's national women's football team, the Indomitable Lionesses, and in the female leagues around the country that feed the national team with top talent. Yolanthe, one of the association's founders, had played on the national team. She led the association during Project ACT. Yolanthe told me that when she played on the national team, male coaches routinely extorted sexual favors from female players. The coaches threatened to claim certain players were lesbians on national radio, to ensure these women succumbed to pressure. The coaches stole players' bonuses as another means of coercing and abusing them. Sharing their experiences of violence and desiring to protect their younger sisters, compelled Yolanthe and several teammates to action. Over a period of 12 years, Yolanthe and the other former players became prominent national advocates against gender-based violence (directed at cisgender women of all sexual orientations) and spokespeople for the rights of cisgender women and girls in sport. The association gradually expanded their work to address women's sexual health needs, including HIV-focused efforts.

When Guy, Emil, and Richard approached her in 2018 about their plans for Project ACT, Yolanthe did not hesitate to commit her association to assist in documenting stigma and discrimination perpetrated against gay and bisexual men and transgender women in Yaoundé's largest HIV outpatient clinical settings. The two associations possessed common concerns, values, and goals. They had similar origin stories, as associations that formed among people with a shared identity to battle abuse and discrimination. Both sought to promote human rights. Both sought to address vulnerability to HIV infection. Both possessed staff and constituents who were sexual minorities and subject to prejudiced treatment in health care settings. As an association advocating for women, Yolanthe and her colleagues no doubt recognized that women share many vulnerabilities with the communities at the heart of Project ACT, communities that are also violated by the social power accorded to cisgender, heterosexual men.

Yolanthe contributed two of her association staff members to the project and sent them off to the 2-day mystery patient training provided by Positive Generation. As is the local custom, those two staff offered a restitution training to everyone else.[2] In this way, the honor of being chosen for this special mission of serving as mystery patients was repaid to the colleagues who were not selected for it; those unchosen colleagues got to learn how to fulfill the mystery patient role. In the spring of 2019, one of the two chosen staff left his position. Yolanthe took his place, becoming a mystery patient herself. Because Project ACT focused on the experiences of gay, bisexual, and other men who have sex with men, and transgender women, when she made her visits to area health care facilities, Yolanthe chose to present herself as male. A petite and slender woman with a lithe athletic frame and long box braids, she adopted the dress typical of young men. Between July 2019 and January 2020, Yolanthe made six mystery patient visits, coordinating with her colleague, Andre, to be sure that they did not appear at the same facility at the same time on the same day. At each facility, she sought an HIV test or sexual health counseling, as instructed. She gave close attention to events and how she was treated at every phase of these visits. She took note of the staff who were rude or impatient, violated her right to privacy, asked her repeatedly if she were a man or a woman, or simply ignored her. She made a mental record of the open logbook of patients' names and HIV test results sitting in plain view of her, its pages easy to read from where she had been instructed to sit. She committed details to memory, such as the absence of HIV posttest counseling on one occasion and of a nurse who broadcast her HIV test result to a room full of other patients on another. She memorized the surprisingly positive experiences, too. She made scratch notes in the cab on the way back to the office, scribbling furiously as the crowded yellow Toyota bumped and swerved over pavement as it gave way to rutted clay. She wrote up her notes in detail once she arrived back at her desk. Once she had completed the standardized form, checking off boxes for each of 11 indicators, and written her narrative account of her visit, she filed her report in the centralized online data repository.

Some scholars argue that identity-based organizations, like the partners to Project ACT, are wise to seek allies at intersections of identity (see, for example, Curtin et al., 2016). Activism to address shared structural disadvantages can be promoted by focusing on points of intersection. Advocating at intersections might exert greater pressure and build community power. As Yolanthe's and her association's participation in Project ACT suggests, vital allies are not necessarily in positions of social privilege themselves, even if they do not share the disadvantaged identity of principal focus. She and the other activists in her association were disenfranchised by the same heteropatriarchal system that oppresses gay and bisexual men and transgender women. Her association's commitment to participate in Project ACT was compelled by the obvious parallels between women's marginalization and the marginalization of gay, bisexual, and other men who have sex with men and of transgender women. Violence, abuse, and discrimination suffered by sexual minority women also spurred her allyship. Lesbians, gay and bisexual men, and transgender people face common oppressions and suffer the same gendered forms of powerlessness. Gender-based violence is one point of their intersecting experiences.

Unsurprisingly, given the dynamics of gender and power (e.g., Connell, 2013; Rosenthal & Levy, 2010), nearly every one of the Project ACT partners employs cisgender women of diverse sexual orientations. Cisgender women are on their boards. Cisgender women are in their volunteer corps. Cisgender women are among their consultants. Many of the Project ACT partners leveraged cisgender women allies to the benefit of the advocacy effort. Another critical reason partnerships form across gender lines is because cisgender women and their concerns are often politically easier to accept and understand—colloquially termed "legibility"—than are sexual minority people and their concerns. This may be especially true in Africa, where cisgender women comprise a large if not the largest proportion of people living with HIV and play crucial roles as activists and leaders. Gender-crossing partnerships also make sense, given what is at the core of both cisgender women's—rights and LGBT—rights global movements—the struggle for bodily autonomy and self-determination.

Additionally, some scholars view homophobia (and transphobia) as extensions of sexism and heterosexism. They, like sexism and misogyny, are socially and institutionally sanctioned tools of force, meant to keep heteronormative gender roles in place, reinforcing male power and privilege over cisgender and transgender women, and gender nonconforming individuals.

Intersectoral Allyship

The Project ACT partners perceived the kinds of partnerships exemplified by Positive Generation, REPMASCI, and Yolanthe's association of women in sport as significant because each reflected collaboration between LGBT community-led identity-based organizations and other civil society organizations in national settings in which these horizontal partnerships are challenging to form. Yet these partnerships are, by their nature, intrasectoral relationships among civil society organizations of similar mission, size, budget, and operating culture. They are, in some fundamental sense, partnerships among the like-minded. Advocacy organizations, as Mitchell et al. note, require intersectoral allies, too (2020). Strategically establishing relationships within government, business, and other sectors and becoming adept at interacting with these non-like-minded entities can aid advocacy organizations in achieving their desired impact. Nearly all Project ACT actors pursued intersectoral collaborators, too. The intersectoral collaborations that the Project ACT partners formed were varied in nature. Several had the purpose of cultivating champions who could elevate the importance of eliminating barriers to HIV care on the priority list of local decision makers in health care and government. Two quite different intersectoral allies illustrate these kinds of intersectoral collaborators.

In Zimbabwe, the Sexual Rights Centre convinced the matrons[3] of the two health facilities they intended to target—a centrally located clinic run by Population Services International and the regional municipal hospital known locally as Mpilo—to identify a small number of colleagues from each of these facilities who might be willing to undergo specialized training in developing advocacy workplans with the idea that, once trained, these staff would be better prepared to champion the issues of access to care within their facilities. These workers would also receive sensitization training, such as the one in which Promise provided testimony (Chapter 5). Both matrons were already interested in figuring out how to serve "key populations" better because the Zimbabwean Ministry of Health was quietly pushing for nationwide progress in meeting the HIV health care needs of these groups in terms of ART provision. Engaging with Project ACT, as one of the two matrons put it, "clarified their purpose."

Many of the health care workers that the matrons convinced to become part of Project ACT were other nurses. Mpilo and Population Services International each operate on a nurse-driven model of care. Mpilo is also among the primary institutions providing nursing education in the region. Registration and payment clerks and other frontline staff comprised the rest of the group the matrons recruited. I met with the matrons and four of these health care workers in 2019. In our meeting, the workers described their interest in health care professions as "a calling"; it was their purpose in life to "help and heal." These workers' noble view of their professional obligations primed their willingness to engage in the Project ACT alliance. In our discussion, they said that they had considered the role religious and other personal values ought to play in health care as part of their decision making about joining in the advocacy work. Notably, they spoke about the potential for personal values to interfere with a health care worker's fulfillment of their calling. They said it was their duty to the public to prioritize help, healing, and service to all over any other values. As one put it:

> When it comes to key populations, values can be disabling for assisting people. People see gay people as demonic. Workers preach societal norms of ignorance that they are animals and should be castigated. That means they [health care workers] become spiritually malnourished.

The matrons and the health care workers recognized their perspective was of the minority. They knew they risked creating friction with their colleagues and deeply offending some of them. But they viewed stigma and discrimination in health care provision as violations of their professional code of nursing ethics. Obeisance to those ethics and to service, not to judgement, convinced them of the importance of getting involved and taking the risk of workplace ostracism.

The health care workers participated in a multiple-day training on advocacy provided by the MPact country lead. They characterized the training as providing them with an entirely new way to see their workplaces. As we talked, they excitedly generated innovative ideas for advocacy actions to target their workplaces, the training still fresh in their minds. Finding creative ways to inject training in affirming care into the nursing school curriculum was among their ideas. In addition to completing the advocacy training, they agreed to participate in quarterly meetings with the Sexual Rights Centre staff and the young men working as peer mobilizers (Chapter 5). In these meetings, they reviewed the ongoing data collected by the peer mobilizers on gay and bisexual men's patient experiences in their facilities. Together with young men, they developed redress plans prompted by specific instances of stigma and discrimination and by general patterns observed in the data. At the urging of the country lead and with his help, the Sexual Rights Centre convinced the leadership of both PSI and Mpilo to support the community–health care worker partnership with a standing Memorandum of Understanding, cementing the intersectoral alliance.

In Cameroon, Affirmative Action pursued relationships with key actors in the government sector. In their case, the relationships included government leaders within and outside the system of public health. Notably, the organization succeeded in convincing Cameroon's Secretary General of the National Commission on Human Rights and Freedoms to sit on the board and engage in select aspects of Project ACT. The Secretary General was appointed to her role in 2014 by Cameroon's president, Paul Biya, an authoritarian leader who has led the country since 1982. Although many in the international human rights community consider the Commission a weak institution with little true authority, the Commission's charter specifies its role as conducting inquiries into reported human rights violations, inspecting the country's penitentiaries, proposing policy measures to advance human rights, and liaising with civil society institutions throughout the country. As the most highly placed national figure charged with advancing human rights, the Secretary General's engagement with Affirmative Action was in many respects a natural step toward fulfilling the Commission's charge. She also had leverage in and connections that could benefit the advocacy work laid out in Project ACT. In my meetings with her over the course of the project, she repeatedly expressed the view that her primary role is that of a national advocate. "Complaining," she told me, "leads to action." As a skilled politician, she saw her involvement with Affirmative Action and her contributions to Project ACT as both necessary and well-timed:

> Identity groups work together and among themselves. That was justified originally. Now we need to join with the general population to promote better understanding in order to end stigma, discrimination, and violence and bring an end to suffering. We have to foster a progressive understanding. This cannot exist in our society without sensitization.

The Secretary General, despite how much of her time was occupied with overseeing investigations of gross human rights violations in the country's ongoing civil war, made sure that she was present at key project events. Her alliance increased the project's visibility and brought others to the Project ACT table. She signed certificates of accomplishment for each of the original mystery patients and each of the partnering identity organizations. Other officials joined her in lending their signatures to the certificates.

A second type of intersectoral collaboration focused simply on bridge building to government and other sectors. This type of bridge building was pursued to better understand the challenges in the sector and develop goodwill. Bridge building led to the identification of novel advocacy targets and to opportunities for reciprocal assistance. J-FLAG's bridge-building work stands out for its intersectoral focus, which included building relationships with educators, business leaders, religious leaders, police, and members of Parliament. This intersectoral orientation is part of J-FLAG's basic approach to advocacy and advancing human rights in all domains of Jamaican life. For other Project ACT partners, HIV was a much more central aspect of their work, often by necessity (Chapter 2).

The J-FLAG staff hosted a series of intimate conversations in which people from different sectors gathered to talk, share a meal, and identify how they might help one another. The meeting I observed of teachers (Chapter 5) was part of this series. In the discussion with teachers, the teachers described the sanctions against teachers that prevent them from intervening on behalf of sexual and gender minority students. They made it plain that it is not just students who are attacked and silenced in school.

Teachers are bullied in ways that make it difficult to stand up for sexual and gender minority children. Deep-seated fear that defending stigmatized children might be used against them and jeopardize their livelihood stops them from acting to make change in their schools. They strike a balance, they said, between giving extra time and attention to LGBT students—especially those whose educational progress had been harmed by being shuttled from school to school—and shouldering the risk that their attention will be misinterpreted. Male teachers, they said, must be especially worried about their attention being perceived as predatory. As their conversation evolved, the advocacy targets in schools came into sharp focus for the J-FLAG staff. The teachers identified lack of workplace protections, principal support, and psychological resources for teachers. Other building-bridges conversations produced a similar result, laying out a roadmap for joint action.

Conclusion

One key to successfully engaging allies lies in the ability to grasp their interests, motivations, and needs, and to situate the benefits of alliances within that frame. Such framing is especially important in contexts in which there is little incentive to form alliances with socially stigmatized (and criminalized) people. Collaboration and allyship pose risks to both partners, although those risks differ. For the Project ACT partners, forming close alliances with actors in the very systems they hoped to change had the potential to co-opt rather than aid their efforts. For the intersectoral allies, they risked staining their reputations and incurring stigma for choosing to partner with LGBT activists. Why take the risk of championing LGBT causes?

In the case of mainstream allies like REPMASCI and Positive Generation, these actors' missions included preventing HIV and improving the state of health care for people living with HIV. Contributing to Project ACT was entirely consistent with and could contribute to fulfillment of their missions. REPMASCI's leaders, who understood that credible reporting on HIV required accurate coverage of the issues concerning "key populations," needed allies such as Alternative Côte d'Ivoire so they could learn about sexual orientation and gender identity and expression. Through a partnership with Alternative Côte d'Ivoire, they could become more skilled in addressing the issues. They could secure access to sexual and gender minority constituents for their journalism. They could become known to the community as a safe and trustworthy media resource. In Cameroon, Positive Generation's leaders were eager to hone their watchdog approach to capture data on access to treatment for "key population" subgroups. Project ACT permitted them to gain their sea legs. If they could pioneer this kind of data collection, they could fill a chasm in the national accountability surveillance system for entities funded by PEPFAR and the Global Fund, upping their national profile and their competitiveness for new funding.

For the intersectoral actors, like the nurses of Zimbabwe and journalists of Côte d'Ivoire, bringing practice closer to professional imperatives compelled their engagement. The Project ACT partners, including their intrasectoral allies, appealed directly to those professional ideals and codes of ethical standards. The handful of journalists in Côte d'Ivoire who agreed to position stories did so because they saw it as consistent with the ideals of their profession. It aligned with their responsibility to disseminate impartial information to the public: "It is my job to put out information. We must treat this seriously. I pushed to get this [information] on the air. It went to my sense of professionalism as a journalist to do it," one journalist explained. He went on to describe being stigmatized by his colleagues for insisting that his station manager allow him to air three programs on LGBT people and their right to health care. His sense of professional integrity trumped his colleagues' stigmatization.

The shared benefits of allying with an association such as Yolanthe's, and with the many other community-led identity associations and organizations that were part of Project ACT, are easiest to identify. Breaking down barriers to care and attacking gendered forms of oppression and violence served the needs of their organizations and constituents. Intersectional allies had the opportunity to gain something to achieve their missions, including developing new expertise, acquiring data, forging new relationships, and demonstrating their own ability to responsibly carry subcontracts. Most importantly, by acting together in coordination, they harnessed the collective power necessary to hold the attention of more powerful local actors, to inch their agenda forward, and to give the issues that drove their partnerships greater visibility than any one of them might achieve by going it alone.

7

Knocked Back on Our Heels

On the night the Rainbow House burned to rubble and ash, more was lost than a building. Before fire incinerated it, the Rainbow House had offered its inhabitants sanctuary in a private tropical oasis. Behind its solid, unmarked iron gate, the compound's interior lay in shade, fringed with palmetto palms, wild limes, and black mango trees laden with fruit. Flowering shrubs, succulents, and medicinal plants grew in profuse clusters alongside the compound's interior walls. Decades before the fire, a former resident of the house had planted an apple tree in the yard, a prized memento of a trip to the United States. It stood majestically in an overgrown patch of garden behind the home, thriving in the unfamiliar tropical conditions. When the work became too much and the crowded conditions inside the modest domicile called for a moment of solitude, people frequently escaped from the small house to sit outdoors under the shelter of the trees or laze on the front porch. The yard was a place of self-care. The wall surrounding the home shielded its residents from the hostile and unfriendly. Except for an occupant of the multistory building next door who might occasionally glance down into the compound and observe young people clustered together in animated conversation, twirling in the sandy soil, swatting badminton birdies back and forth, or hunching over their cellphones, few would know that this unexceptional dwelling on Stanton Terrace housed Jamaica's foremost LGBT human rights organization.

Inside the structure, in the worn entry foyer, used as a reception area, a small library of LGBT history books, including rare first editions, lined the shelves of a cupboard. Newspaper clippings highlighting key moments in local LGBT history sat on display on a side table. In the interior rooms, desks were jammed together in an untidy jumble. In one room, the desks were packed so tightly it was difficult to move in and around them, let alone pull up an extra chair to work alongside a colleague. The sole bathroom in the house served double duty—toilet and storage—its bathtub brimming with supplies. A set of posters documenting J-FLAG's history and honoring its founders sat askew in the tub. Staff had created these posters for display at an event celebrating J-FLAG's 20th anniversary held just 3 weeks before the fire. Nearly all these artifacts were destroyed in the blaze. The fire burnt to cinders every financial record, the main J-FLAG server, the computers, and most of the office furniture. Water from the futile attempt to save the building ruined what the fire did not destroy. Official estimates are that 90% of the building and its content was lost in the blaze. Staff were able to rescue little of what had survived intact. Anything worth rescuing

Breaking Barriers. Robin Lin Miller and George Ayala, Oxford University Press. © Oxford University Press 2024.
DOI: 10.1093/oso/9780197647684.003.0008

was stolen long before the staff were permitted by fire investigators to pass through the iron gate for the last time to retrieve what might be salvaged.[1]

The Rainbow House had been a place of gathering, of organizing, of mobilizing, of strategizing, of sanctuary, and of remembering. It was more difficult to bask in a sense of community with the staff flung wide and far across Kingston. Locating a property owner willing to rent to the LGBT organization and who could offer them affordable, adequate space in a safe enough neighborhood proved difficult. Ten months after the fire, J-FLAG had yet to identify a new permanent home. The staff continued to squeeze itself into a too small, barely furnished temporary office space in an office building in New Kingston. They slumped in beanbag chairs on the floor, laptops balanced on their knees.

Access to space outside of Rainbow House had been a perennial issue for the J-FLAG staff. They were veterans of being denied space, which only added to the wound inflicted by the house's loss. Staff could rely on just a handful of New Kingston hotels to host events. Many venue owners simply refused the group access to their properties. The staff had grown weary of venue owners cancelling events at the last minute, which was especially common outside of Kingston. Proprietors' anxieties rose intolerably as they reckoned with the thought of a large gathering of queer people, so they chose to back out of the deal. "Venue owners cancel. We had an event cancelled at the last minute because the poster created too much visibility for the venue owner. We also need to be sure venues are safe for the community," Jada explained from the well of her beanbag chair. Ironically, an event she and Akoni hoped that I (Robin) might attend with the staff was cancelled by the venue owner a day or two after Jada and I spoke. Finding a friendly enough proprietor to rent J-FLAG new space was not the only pressing problem Akoni had to address in recovering from the fire. Reconstituting the organization's financial history would take him the better part of 2019, the same months that comprised the peak of activity on Project ACT. The retrieval effort, coupled with the protracted process of raising the capital necessary to replace the material items the organization had lost, proved a major source of distraction from his regular work of onboarding and supervising staff, and overseeing J-FLAG's robust portfolio of national advocacy. Fires never come at opportune times, but for Akoni, it simply could not be worse. Jaden, his right-hand assistant, was on leave overseas for the year to earn an advanced degree.

The fire that destroyed the Rainbow House was but one among many acute and chronic challenges that tested the toughness of a Project ACT partner. Disasters like the Rainbow House fire might impede the project's advocacy work, a worrisome problem given the project's ambitious nature and its blistering timeline. The work in Jamaica had barely begun when the fire halted the staff in their tracks and dispersed them across the city. Dymond had organized and hosted only three community conversations (Chapter 5) when the fire caught. Candice, the policy expert hired to work alongside Dymond in Jaden's place, had been onboarded just 5 months before the house went up in smoke. She was in the preliminary stages of determining how to move an agenda forward that would serve the project's goals. But she had already decided J-FLAG's playful, "cliquish" culture did not suit her. She planned to quit, which, after the fire, she did.

This chapter examines how the Project ACT partners responded to adverse and unexpected events while implementing their advocacy activities. In every setting, a wide range of challenges emerged: from security threats to political upheaval, to disaster, to the overwhelming stress of addressing violence and human rights abuses. Some disturbances were tied closely to the ongoing work, whereas others resulted from increased tensions and uncertainties of the larger political, economic, and cultural context. Still others resulted from oversights and miscalculations in planning. This chapter will lay out how these occurrences impacted the ongoing advocacy and identifies the resources and principles in action that assisted the partners to weather challenges.

Throughout Project ACT's implementation, events entirely beyond their control knocked partners back on their heels. Disasters large and small and shifting political dynamics occurred in every country, reshaping the project's backdrop and disrupting partners' plans. Adaptation to changing circumstances and acute catastrophic episodes may be especially important for community-led organizations like those in Project ACT, as they operate from a marginal social, political, and economic position in even the best of conditions. An organization's ability to rebound in the face of contextual and institutional challenges is key to its survival and to the success of its activities. Organizations must not only prepare for and adapt to inevitable disturbances and trials but also learn from them, transforming how they approach their work (Duchek, 2020).

Barasa and colleagues (2018) term the ability to grow in the face of chronic and acute challenges "adaptative resilience." Duchek suggests a resilient organization is characterized by its ability to anticipate and prepare for undesirable events and circumstances, cope and problem-solve when undesired events occur, and learn in the wake of disturbances. Broadly speaking, the literature suggests that three types of resources enable organizations to withstand inevitable shocks: material resources, social resources, and reflective capability. Whether and how these resources enable LGBT community-led organizations to rise in the face of adversity is poorly understood, especially in national contexts in which government-sponsored harassment is routine, and organizations are supported in their work principally by partners from governments and foundations based outside the region. Through an examination of Project ACT's challenges, we explore the role each of these types of resources played in responding to diverse challenges.

Material Resources

To the extent that adequate material resources matter when threats to an organization and its activities occur, the Project ACT partners operated at a tremendous disadvantage. Material resources were in short supply. No partner possessed cash reserves to manage a situation like the Rainbow House fire or the spiraling decline of the Zimbabwean economy. Rather, the Project ACT partners survived on little. Indeed, limited financing and material resources were high on the list of chronic strains that restricted how the partners could respond to unanticipated turns in events throughout the project period. Among the four organizations we followed intensively throughout the project, J-FLAG was the wealthiest among them. Akoni reported that for the fiscal year prior to Project ACT, the organization functioned on an annual budget of just over US$900,000, funds which supported the staff of 14, excluding its security guard, advocacy activities and training expenses, and paid the rent at Rainbow House in Kingston's expensive real estate market. Penya calculated the Sexual Rights Centre's total budget for the fiscal year preceding Project ACT at US$729,401; its staff, ex-cluding the volunteered labor of its collective leaders and its full-time groundskeeper, comprised 13 people. It rented out two homes, using one for staff offices. The other provided office space to its collective leaders, meeting space for programming, and an outdoor space where staff, constituents, and guests spend time together and gather for tea and communal meals. According to Guy, Affirmative Action's annual budget totaled US$433,851. At the start of Project ACT, the association supported the largest staff of all—27 people—and was the only one with decentralized operations in mul-tiple locations spread throughout the country, a potentially wise strategy for a sexual minority-led organization in a criminalizing country. Affirmative Action rented out a small former home in Yaoundé as its headquarters, stuffing staff members elbow to elbow into cramped former bedrooms that now served as communal offices.[2] Claude, although he expressed uncertainty that he had his figures correct, indicated that he thought Alterative Côte d'Ivoire operated on a modest annual budget of US$180,654. At the start of Project ACT, he estimated 16 people were on the payroll part- or full-time. MPact's annual budget the year before Project ACT was US$3.6 million, although it channeled US$1.7 million of that amount to community-led partners around the globe. The remaining money supported its 13 staff members, operating expenses, rent of a small one-room office in downtown Oakland, California, and the expense of constant travel and hosting of the transnational convenings that are essen-tial to its global organizing, advocacy, and capacity-building mission.

The funding climate for the Project ACT partners is treacherous and made more severe by declining national investments in HIV and limited sources of financial sup-port for advocacy (Chapter 2). Except for MPact, and to a lesser extent J-FLAG, the partners described their funding as focused on discrete donor-driven projects, most of which were tied to narrow aspects of HIV service delivery along the continuum of care. PEPFAR and the Global Fund provided the bulk of that support, with lesser amounts provided from sources such as the Canadian, Dutch, and French govern-ments. Partners characterized funding for programs specific to sexual and gender minorities as quite rare, and especially funding to address stigma, discrimination, and human rights abuses, which are of high priority to the local community. "I don't see any grant to support MSM more than MPact," Mbuso observed as we sat in the dark in Penya's office. His colleague, Peter, described available funding as keeping

organizations "stuck" in providing a limited array of services, such as condom distribution and HIV testing. "Mostly other projects, they focus more on the health to be
required, access to medicines, access to commodities and all that," he explained.

The perennial need to piece together project funding to support a minimum core
staff often pushed the Project ACT organizations to operate beyond their human resource capacity. They pursued projects that might strain the staff simply to ensure
they had sufficient resources to cover a minimum of personnel. Relying on project-
based funding to cover the salaries for core staff contributed to layoffs when projects ended, leading to an accompanying loss of expertise. The constant scrambling
and unpredictable nature of funding was a problem to which none of the Project
ACT organizations was immune. It was simply too hard to forecast which resource
scenario—abundance or drought—was on the immediate horizon. During the unexpected or rare windfall period, new projects fell onto the shoulders of overstretched
staff. The MPact staff found themselves in precisely this position at the start of Project
ACT (Chapter 3). A fear expressed by partners on each of my visits was that the
funding for Project ACT would end just as the work gained traction, leading to layoffs
and loss of momentum.

Project-oriented funding made it especially difficult to maintain a depth of staff in
policy and advocacy. As Akoni noted in our first conversation after the fire, "it is hard
to support policy officers and those who are dedicated exclusively to policy work."
Moreover, service delivery required hiring staff with different capabilities. Seasoned
activists have honed their skills in legal and policy analysis, advocacy strategy, diplomacy, and other competencies that are fundamental to moving an advocacy agenda
forward. Infrastructure support was uncommon, too. Organizations' material resources were restricted to a project-focused budget, with the bare minimum administrative support staff needed to deal with essential matters such as finance. Some of
the organizations employed a monitoring and evaluation staff person, but as is too
often the case, none were trained in monitoring or evaluation or a cognate specialization. Most also had other duties. Keeping track of attendance at training sessions
and workshops, counting the number of condoms distributed and the administration
and results of HIV tests, and monitoring other donor-determined indicators formed
the bulk of their activities. They monitored often and evaluated seldom, if ever. None
of the Project ACT partners had a development officer. Few engaged in non-project-
focused fundraising campaigns. All had limited (if any) discretionary funding. One
of the reasons J-FLAG lost its financial records in the fire was because, lacking robust
administrative and information technology resources, the policy staff had been gradually scanning 20 years of paper records into a database as their time permitted. They
had made little progress when the building turned into ashes.

The Project ACT budgets, too, were of little help when faced with trouble. The
amount of money each partner received was paltry in comparison to the work most
had proposed. Budget limitations, for example, were the sole reason so few members
of the gay and bisexual constituencies of the Sexual Rights Centre could participate in
the LILO workshops (Chapter 5). Gay and bisexual men are estimated to number at

least 800 in Bulawayo.[3] The budget supported offering the training to 30 people. Young men complained (Chapter 5) that so few in the community had the privilege to attend the workshop because of limited funds. In Cameroon, the advocacy work relied on two tactics, one of which was to document stigma and discrimination in health care settings using mystery patient methods (Bober et al., 2019; Daouk-Öyry et al., 2018; McGinn & Irani, 2019). The mystery patients were drawn from community-led organizations. The mystery patient role was new for them all. But budget constraints led Positive Generation, Affirmative Action's collaborator (Chapter 6), to compress what would have ordinarily been a 5-day training for mystery patients filled with role-play rehearsals and practice, into just 2 days. Shortchanging mystery patients' training due to funding constraints led to initial data quality problems that required swift corrective action on the part of Positive Generation. On the first attempt at data collection, Positive Generation found it necessary to deploy their veteran data collectors to make up for observations they believed were too poorly conducted to use.

Mystery patients had also not been provided funds with which to seek actual services. They had instead been instructed to inquire about certain services but told not to pay for the booklet that would permit them to get beyond the initial registration process. By not purchasing a booklet, the methodology was, by default, focused on rooting out price gouging and whether services that should be available were in fact made available, consistent with the original focus of Positive Generation. Mystery patient reports of stigma and discrimination were therefore limited to whether they were provided with accurate cost information, whether they were stonewalled at the initial stages of the patient registration process, and whether they were exposed to abuse, degrading remarks, unkind stares, and the like at the main entry points to services. They did not obtain information on stigma and discrimination in the context of actual exams for real health conditions, as did mystery patients in the other Project ACT countries. This frustrated them. As Thea, a transgender mystery patient, explained to me, "We expected to go further, but we didn't have enough money. 10,000 XAF just covered transportation." In my interviews, activists often recounted instances of the humiliating treatment their constituents had endured in the context of an examination. By not attempting to obtain actual care, including specialized care, the approach that served Positive Generation so well over time failed to capture stigma and discrimination in areas of unique need for gay and bisexual men and transgender women, notably penile and anal health, and gender-affirming care. Mystery patients and the leaders of the identity organizations I spoke with were dissatisfied with the approach for this reason, especially given the serious condyloma epidemic among gay and bisexual men in Cameroon at the time. One matron estimated that 40%–50% of the gay and bisexual men in her clinic's care presented with rectal condyloma. Many of the stories I heard from advocates of humiliating patient–provider interactions concerned the diagnosis and treatment of rectal condyloma.

Many factors led to a mismatch between resources and ambitions. Struggling for funding and having to compete against professionalized nongovernment organizations (Chapter 2) had schooled the organizations in overpromising. The long and difficult negotiations between MPact and the LGBT Fund over the project itself (Chapter 3) contributed to underfunding an effort for which there were exceedingly high hopes for what might be accomplished quickly, despite the immense scope of the work and diverse country settings. Moreover, the project's scope of work was never appropriately revised to account for the sizable fee UNAIDS charged to pass the money from the United States government to the LGBT Fund (Chapter 3). MPact's decision to distribute funds in equal amounts to every partner, rather than make country-level budgetary decisions as a function of what was needed to carry out the proposed advocacy workplan, also contributed to monetary challenges. Through its equal treatment, MPact provided too many resources to some partners relative to what they intended to do, considering local costs and their ability to absorb the funds quickly. This left others, such as the Sexual Rights Centre and Affirmative Action, to pinch and scrape and, at times cut corners, accomplishing less than they could have otherwise. "Distributing equal amounts of money across countries did not work," one of the MPact country leads observed in our final interview. "We should have done a deeper analysis of each project's requirements."

Resource strains were exacerbated, too, by mismatches in activities and budgets that arose from some organizations' limited skills in translating their workplans into budgets. Some organizations requested less than they required, failing to budget for a line item. Although MPact remedied these oversights and miscalculations as best they could, the small size of the overall project budget limited how much remedy they could offer. MPact's part of the funds supported the following: the time of the MPact country leads and the other staff who provided project support, the costs for MPact staff to travel to countries, the costs of convening everyone involved in the project at the two multiday cross-learning face-to-face meetings—one in Cambodia (Chapter 4) and a second in Rwanda—and the fees for engaging the services of six translators. From what was left over, MPact partially funded the cost of evaluation. At the level of the entire project portfolio, MPact, too, had insufficient resources to cover costs matching its aspirations.

Addressing the Impact of Limited Monetary Resources

In the context of limited financial resources, J-FLAG's ability to continue its functioning after the fire depended in no small part on the willingness of its allies, including the local UNAIDS office with which the group had a strong relationship, and peer organizations such as Caribbean Vulnerable Communities, to allow J-FLAG staff to use their meeting rooms open-endedly. It also benefited from allies such as MPact mobilizing and providing material support. MPact rebudgeted immediately to provide US$10,000 in emergency funds to J-FLAG for urgent needs, such as replacing its incinerated computers. Leveraging the support of allies allowed the Jamaican team to remain focused on their mission. Equally important, the flexible nature of the project permitted partners to pursue a diverse set of advocacy tactics and to develop and support nascent transgender organizations, rather than narrowly bound their efforts around a single advocacy strategy, tactic, and target. This flexibility proved key to J-FLAG's ability to emerge from the fire while still progressing on Project ACT. The Jamaican team had conceived of its work as progressing down multiple pathways. When their focus on national policy was set aside so that Akoni could address the fire's aftermath, Dymond's work progressed uninterrupted on other fronts; her work took center stage. J-FLAG benefited in the face of this unanticipated disaster from conceiving of Project ACT as a set of complementary activities carried out by several individuals, each of whom were accorded a high degree of autonomy. Broadly speaking, investing in a diversity of advocacy actions averted the need for a near total pause in their activity. It also proved key to their successes (Chapter 8).

The Sexual Rights Centre had started to resist allowing donors' prerogatives to guide their sense of priorities. "The service work is donor driven and must be done because that is where the funds are," Penya explained. "The advocacy is community driven. In the past, SRC took any funds uncritically. We are moving away from that now and will pass up on funds that don't align with the advocacy agenda we are now refining." During Project ACT, reliable access to money, electricity, and fuel proved significant obstacles to the Sexual Rights Centre's work. The staff endured multiple consecutive days each week without electricity, lasting from about 5 a.m. to after 11 p.m. Access to diesel fuel to run the office's generators or move around the city was unreliable. In January 2019, Zimbabwe, experienced nationwide riots prompted by a surprise 130% increase in the price of fuel, amid widespread diesel and food shortages (Burke, 2019; Human Rights Watch, 2019c). To regain control over the situation, the Zimbabwean government deployed its security forces and shut down the Internet nationwide. Citizens were ordered to stay home and remain indoors, shuttering businesses, banks, and schools and, by a coincidence of poor timing, trapping Mohan, the country lead, in a modest lodge for the duration of what was meant to be his inaugural week in the country working with the Sexual Rights Centre staff. When I visited the Centre 2 weeks after the riots, military checkpoints remained along the main roads into town. Government crackdowns, routine electricity load-sharing shutoffs, fuel shortages, and rampant inflation continued throughout the year, dashing the optimism and hope the Centre staff felt when President Emmerson Mnangagwa first succeeded Robert Mugabe in 2017. Mugabe was known as an enemy of LGBT people. Mnangagwa had seemed more temperate in his public statements, at least so far. During their strategic planning retreat, held the week of my postriot visit, the uncertainty that the staff and their countrypeople now faced cast a long shadow over their plans for 2019. Come May, the government cracked down hard on human rights workers, arresting several at Harare's airport upon their return from meetings abroad, prompting the Sexual Rights Centre staff to operate on high alert and low profile.

In June 2019, Zimbabwe's government abruptly introduced a new Zimbabwean dollar. Overnight, foreign currency was no longer legal tender, although the country had relied on the US dollar as its primary form of tender for several years.[4] The new Zimbabwean dollar was worth little relative to US currency. It remained impossible to buy fuel without US dollars. The abrupt shift in policy accelerated intense hyper-inflation, which by all estimates, exceeded 500% by the end of 2019. At one point, money simply dried up and could not be obtained through the bank. Mbuso noted the staff repeatedly devised work-around systems with every shift in monetary policy and access to currency to ensure that community mobilizers could receive stipends and subsidies for transportation and supplies. The staff cycled rapidly through cell-phone payment systems, distributing US dollars, and point systems, depending upon which made the most sense in the moment. The advocacy kept going because of the creative solutions devised through ongoing teamwork and discussion, and through a willingness to work without financial support.

Social Resources

As Project ACT's partners struggled to launch and implement their work, they received help from local networks (Chapter 6) and benefitted from MPact's broad reach. Over its history, MPact staff maintained a regular presence in global efforts to ensure community input into the development of the Country Operational Plans (COPs) that serve as national guides to the HIV response. MPact routinely prepared community-led organizations for contributing to their national planning process. Another focus of MPact's advocacy work involved applying pressure to ensure that gay and bisexual men's organizations were chosen to participate in national and regional convenings (see Chapter 2). Indeed, one goal of Project ACT in Burundi was to secure a seat at the COP planning table for a LGBT community-led group. Positioning and preparing gay and bisexual men's organizations to operate in these arenas was a priority driving the MPact staff to log thousands of airline miles each year and guaranteeing that MPact's personnel were known around the world to country-level staff in Ministries of Health and to UNAIDS, PEPFAR, and Global Fund officials at global, regional, and national levels. Among the less visible but impactful ways in which MPact staff assisted partners through frustrating obstacles, such as a myriad of unanswered emails and unreturned phone calls from mainstream officials, was to leverage their network of global relationships on the partners' behalf.

In preparing for the project, several of the partners had secured promises from critical government actors to support the work of the project. And just as the project began in earnest, as so often occurs, these individuals left their positions. In República Dominicana, the government restructured the Ministry of Health and its programs. The Ministry of Health leadership turned over during the restructuring, which led to a cascade of other personnel departures. Amigos Siempre Amigos's advocacy work-plan depended entirely on the verbal agreements and collaboration of key individuals who had left the Ministry during this transition. They found themselves obliged to reestablish a relationship with the Ministry and resecure commitments from its new leadership. This, coupled with the Polyplas factory explosion that closed the nearby clinics where the work was slated to begin,[5] pushed back the implementation of their advocacy efforts in earnest by a year. Using MPact as leverage and having the MPact country lead fly in to attend an initial meeting with key government officials, aided the Dominican team in reinvigorating its relationship with the Ministry. In Cameroon, the head of the country's PEPFAR office left shortly after their cooperation in support of Project ACT had been secured. Gaining the attention of the new country director, once they were appointed, took considerable effort and required intervention on the part of the MPact country lead. In cases such as these, the MPact staff were more comfortable and accustomed than the local teams at pushing government actors. In this way, MPact facilitated the ability of local partners to leverage these connections (see Chapter 2). Another element of MPact's strategy for ensuring that partners' efforts were visible to local officials was the routine practice of sending MPact country leads or me (Robin) on courtesy visits when they were in country. MPact viewed the locally based officials as critical resources for ensuring the safety and security of partners (and of me), in addition to strategically ensuring that officials used their power to remove obstacles to the project's success. These audiences, if nothing else, called attention to the local partner and the urgent nature of their work to improve the community's access to affirming and safe HIV and sexual health care services.

The nature of the relationship that evolved between MPact and the Project ACT partners factored heavily in how partners understood MPact's contributions to their work and in their tolerance of MPact's missteps and limitations. Partners perceived MPact as open to hearing about their obstacles, trials, and uncertainties and as available to provide prompt feedback. The quality of these relationships conditioned what MPact brought to each partner's efforts. MPact staff actively nurtured their partners' skills and experiences, facilitated partners' linkages to critical allies and opportunities, remained available and responsive, and succeeded in honoring the dignity, self-worth, knowledge, and expertise of their partners. Partners observed that they were granted the room to engage in problem-solving and to own the project locally. Akoni summed up a common sentiment among the partners. "They gave us the room to ensure our perspective and expertise guided the work.... Partnerships like this allow North-South conversation to occur as distinct from the North instructing the South." Whatever unfulfilled wishes they may have had, none of the partners would trade MPact for another funder.

But Project ACT placed the MPact team under great strain. They took on the work when they were already overwhelmed. They were not always able to live by their own principles, protocols, and aspirations. Partners, no matter how open they were to MPact's mentorship and collaboration, did not feel MPact's presence on the ground as much as they desired. As one partner put it, "Sometimes they just go silent. They disappear on the rudder." For the MPact team too, Project ACT was novel in its demands. Working across three organizational teams—communications, public policy, and public health—was novel. Integrating a prospective participatory evaluation was novel. Like its partners, what was not optimal in its staffing, leadership, budget, and project management was surmounted by the energy, expertise, flexibility, and dedication of staff and the foundation of partnership on which the work rested.

Although the relationships that emerged between MPact and the Project ACT partners were not perfect and partners offered fair criticisms of MPact, as MPact did of its partners, the most troubled relationship in Project ACT proved to be with the LGBT Fund. Operating on a lean base of project-focused funding and with no fat in reserve, the Project ACT organizations relied on timely upfront tranches to pay workers and keep advocacy activities going. This did not always occur, causing suspended activity. Disbursement delays harmed the work at the onset, as it took MPact too long to complete the fiscal audits that preceded setting up electronic payment systems. On another occasion in May 2019, at the height of the project, a delay in disbursement of funds to MPact from the LGBT Fund stopped the work in every country and at MPact itself. The events that led to this delay offer an unfortunate cautionary tale on funder relationships and the power funders have over small community-led groups that operate from a fragile financial position.

Eager to be transparent, MPact's 12-month report to the funder contained more information than the LGBT Fund required. The narrative was chock-full of photographs and peppered with links to country-level products and reports. Inadvertently included among these supplementary pieces of information was a SharePoint link to internal working documents in which the MPact team identified challenges and brainstormed solutions. The project officer clicked on the link and read the confidential materials stored there. His decision to delay the payment was triggered by what he read. A single data placemat[6] from a staff meeting held in April 2019 especially irked him. That placement listed the site visits that had occurred through March. Three of seven countries had been visited by a MPact country lead.[7] He expected every country would have been visited and on more than one occasion. My visits to countries did not count.

MPact was never optimized to meet his expectations. MPact had promised technical support, but not for it to be delivered via regularly occurring, in-person, on-the-ground coaching. In lieu of site visits, MPact had, with his knowledge, rebudgeted to bring everyone together in Cambodia (Chapter 4). They intended to do the same retreat-styled reflection at the project's close because the partners requested it, again rebudgeting to make this possible. MPact found other efficiencies for meeting with partners by piggybacking on regional meetings as part of other projects. Because I was spending time in four of the countries routinely and providing real-time feedback, staff perceived that they had eyes and ears on the ground. For these reasons, the MPact staff did not view it as necessary to have yet made a visit to every partner. The staff later came to view this as a mistake because it would have enhanced their understanding of the context and of each partner organization, but they did not see it that way at the time.[8]

In addition, MPact had engaged in an evaluation solely for themselves, not at the behest of the Fund. This, they believed, was to their credit. MPact perceived the LGBT Fund took no deep interest in evaluation but hoped they might share MPact's perspective that it was an admirable and useful thing to do. It might provide the Fund with a window into the daily rhythms of the advocacy work that the Fund had said they desired to better understand. It would demonstrate MPact's evolution toward improving themselves as a learning organization. It would show them a fit-for-purpose model of evaluation. George and his staff assumed the Fund would find value in learning about community-led advocacy and its potential to contribute to on-the-ground progress in addressing stigma and discrimination. As it turned out, the Fund's interest in evaluation was not at all certain. They had no policy on evaluation. At the time, they had no evaluation officer.

The conflict with the LGBT Fund posed a dilemma for MPact. MPact viewed the LGBT Fund as a partner and ally to the work, not an adversary. MPact had committed itself to transparency, to sharing what it was learning with its funder in real time and to openness about our participatory and transformative evaluation processes and procedures. The MPact staff were therefore flabbergasted that having voluntarily (over)shared what they were fretting over and learning about resulted in a punitive response that imperiled the work at its height. George intervened rapidly and successfully to break the impasse and secure a release of funds, with assistance from me and Nadia. Yet, a month of time that the project could not afford to lose had passed idly by the time tranches eventually reached MPact and, in turn, the partners' bank accounts. During that time, country by country, each team did what they could to prevent the project from sputtering out while they and local partners went unpaid. Their shared vision and commitment to mitigating the inequities that disadvantage their communities kept them going.

Reflective Capacity

MPact's country leads felt they were too rushed over the summer of 2018 to invest in close analysis of the revised workplans partners submitted to them after the Cambodia workshop. The project had to move into the field too quickly (Chapter 3). Despite some plans that were still too ambitious, passive, or undercapacitated, the MPact staff agreed to sign off on them because the clock was loudly ticking. The MPact country leads relied on the hope that the rich quality of their partnerships (and experience in developing relationships with new partners) would allow them to collaborate on continual refinement of the plans as these were being implemented. As one country lead told me later, the MPact practice of holding frequent conversations with partners was his key to ensuring he heard specifics of what was going on. Without that, he said, "You might just be getting the rosy picture of what's happening and not the real challenges." These routine conversations were the opening for brainstorming through obstacles and moments of uncertainty, ongoing iteration, bringing in resources, and helping partners to course-correct to meet their specific goals. Consistent engagement of MPact country leads with their partners through biweekly or monthly reflective check-ins, periodic visits, and our evaluation process served as the main mechanisms for navigating the way forward.

The partners valued this overall strategy because it preserved their autonomy. It allowed them to lead the local work as they thought appropriate to their setting, while also providing them with ways to leverage MPact's expertise, resources, and connections. In many cases, this strategy worked. In organizations such as the Sexual Rights Centre, Penya had purposively moved toward a democratic, deliberative, and inclusive organizational culture to replace the toxic culture she had inherited. For her staff, reflective engagement with MPact was greeted eagerly.[9] Mandala observed that having Mohan make repeated visits was especially meaningful, noting "We've never met many of our partners." Several other partners were similarly welcoming of the opportunity to use their MPact country lead as a sounding board and resource. But to the regret of the MPact country leads, there were also missed opportunities. Sometimes the work in a country had moved too rapidly for the country lead to contribute. Sometimes a country lead's site visit was mistimed. Sometimes the inability to speak the same language got in the way. Sometimes the partner's leadership placed less value on reflection with an external party than MPact had hoped.

At times, the one-on-one reflection sessions with a partner, including reflections on recent evaluation findings, resulted in a simple intervention or minor change in course. For instance, as Dymond steadily worked toward convening a national transgender health conference in Jamaica, she brainstormed ideas with Omar on how to integrate advocacy tactics into the conference. As Mandla and Mbuso started working with young men to mobilize their peers in Zimbabwe, Mohan prompted them to consider obtaining a formal Memorandum of Understanding with the local facilities (Chapter 6). He also came to visit and provided custom advocacy training to local health care champions. As Kofi and Michael attempted to get their Ministry of Health on board in Ghana, Stephen encouraged consideration of how the Ghanian patient charter could be a persuasive tool in their advocacy work. These deliberative conversations and interventions altered the work in each place in ways that may have seemed modest at the time but proved consequential (Chapter 8).

Safety and Security

Among the challenges for which reflection proved critical were those related to safety and security, especially given planning missteps for how safety and security were initially addressed. Given the foreseeable dangers that Project ACT posed and in view of MPact's long-standing emphasis on activist safety and security, the staff had placed safety and security scenario planning on its original agenda for the planning retreat in Cambodia (Chapter 4). Scenario analysis can assist organizations to prepare for and militate against worst-case occurrences. But crafting the contours of safety and security plans was among the items the MPact team limited coverage of in Cambodia to ensure that the Project ACT partners had adequate time and guidance to elaborate their initial workplan ideas (Chapter 4). At the time, this made sense.

For some partners, developing the framework for a formal advocacy workplan was a novel task. Several were new enough to advocacy work that they had never engaged in developing a theory of structural change or conducted analyses of the leverage points in systems of power. Although all possessed advocacy experience, it was often informal or a developing area of competence. Gaston, among the most senior advocates in Cameroon, believed Affirmative Action's staff were advanced beginners in advocacy. He thought they still required training in advanced tools for planning, conducting, and evaluating advocacy. Investing time learning the building blocks of planning campaigns during the Cambodia workshop fit with his view of what staff in his organization needed. "We do not have any training in leading effective advocacy," he said. "What we are doing currently is out of our own experience, not from any training. It's true that we read some books in order to lead advocacy, but these are only readings and not always very accurate." He wanted theory. He wanted strategy. He wanted techniques. Guy agreed with him, noting that the staff knew extraordinarily little about advocacy targeting institutions or in government and public policy arenas. Gaston also pointed out that they had no knowledge of how to evaluate the advocacy they did conduct, a task which at times fell to him. Learning the customized approaches to advocacy evaluation keenly interested him, as it did other partners:

> We also need to know how evaluation of our advocacy is conducted. Because we do not know. As I said, I and my collaborators, we lead advocacy activities to a given point, but at the end of the day we will notice that we are not really able to make an assessment of the advocacy activity to that level.

Other partners were housed in service delivery organizations or felt forced to devote substantial effort to service delivery activities (e.g., HIV testing, outreach, and education) to gain financial support; this is what they were most practiced at developing a workplan around. The novelty of Project ACT set everyone on a tremendous learning curve, but that curve was especially steep for those from organizations for which the project demanded a seismic shift from their ordinary daily repertoire of service provision and normal project planning approaches. Safety and security plan development was not on their list, even if it was an enduring worry. Safety and security plans were also not required in the final workplans or in the line-item budgets. In the end, the only robust safety and security plan developed for the project—and that included the in-kind infrastructure to support its creation and implementation—was for the evaluation.[10] In several countries, the lack of robust funded safety and security plans led to events for which MPact and its partners could have been better prepared.

The Need to Seek Asylum

For several African partners, the project contributed to the possibility that a staff member or constituent would consider pursuing asylum temporarily or permanently. In some cases, the project accelerated processes already unfolding for someone who faced a need to flee. At neither the local nor transnational level was the project fully prepared for this possibility, or at least it was not widely and openly discussed. Nor was the possibility of someone's detention. No local budget included emergency funds to support evacuation or, in the case of an arrest, legal representation. MPact possessed relationships to organizations that specialize in assisting LGBT activists who are in danger to leave their countries quickly and safely. These relationships were not leveraged as a formal resource to the project.

In Burundi, one of the most hostile environments of all, the Project ACT partner focused much of their work on the lack of a well-developed network of registered and nonregistered community-led groups to address LGBT human rights concerns. They also worked on building the nascent infrastructure necessary to document human rights abuses in health care. Documenting violence was also of keen interest. Burundian law limits freedom of expression on sexual orientation and gender identity and restricts the legal registration and operation of organizations focused on sexual orientation. Events and meetings organized by LGBT community-led groups are routinely and quickly shut down by law enforcement. These well-enforced government restrictions on assembly and speech severely limited the ways in which Prosper, Pierre, and Alan could mobilize Burundi's fledgling and clandestine community-led groups around a common agenda. Pierre's initial steps were to travel the country documenting how the legal climate affected community-led groups' ability to organize and conduct basic HIV-related outreach. He traveled because bringing people together in a larger centralized convening was forbidden. As Pierre moved about the country, he was routinely harassed and surveilled by the police. At one point, he contemplated whether he might need to leave the country for his safety, discussing the pros and cons of seeking temporary asylum with Stephen. Pierre's visibility preceded the project, as is generally true of the Project ACT partners and their staff members. Government surveillance of Project ACT activities was predictable.[11]

Safety and security issues also resulted from the nature of the specific advocacy tactics. In Côte d'Ivoire, the Project ACT workplan included training of three LGBT community-led organizations to engage effectively with mainstream media and to produce a series of short videos for distribution to private groups through social media platforms. Several of the videos featured constituents' testimonials of personal harassment, discrimination, and violence. One video proved especially compelling to its viewers, quickly garnering likes, comments, and shares. Its popularity spooked the video's subject, who faced unrelated legal troubles. The subject promptly requested the video be taken offline. Shortly thereafter, the subject relocated to another country for her safety. This incident and concerns about the extent to which the videos followed best practices for protecting the identity of subjects prompted Johnny to urge Alternative Côte d'Ivoire to rebudget and provide additional training for the local organizations, which the organization pursued. Johnny and Greg also went to Abidjan to provide supplementary on-site training in video safety, bringing in a local professional videographer to assist them in coaching the staff. These latter efforts came too late, however, as few videos were left to be produced. In retrospect, the MPact country lead told me he believed it was obvious at the outset that making these kinds of videos was risky, if not pursued with the highest possible safety-informed production quality. Representatives of the three organizations that Alternative Côte d'Ivoire trained believed that, even with their retraining, they were insufficiently prepared to produce high-quality safety-conscious videos, let alone convince people to go on camera to tell their stories. For the MPact country lead, having failed to push each partner to imagine the worst and develop a robust safety plan at the outset troubled him. A key principle of MPact's approach to advocacy practice—safety—had not been given its due.

Protecting Mystery Patients

The challenges with adapting Positive Generation's methodology successfully, noted earlier, also led to safety and security concerns. During my second visit to Cameroon, I interviewed mystery patients and leaders from several of the community-led identity organizations from which the mystery patients were drawn. I also interviewed the staff from Positive Generation for a second time. I learned that the mystery patients, while they valued the training they received from Positive Generation, notably learning about their rights and how things ought to work when they tried to access health care, and the opportunity to be part of the project, were concerned for their psychological safety and physical security.

With so few people acting as mystery patients, mystery patients feared they would be easily found out, especially the transgender mystery patients, invoking backlash and increasing their vulnerability to violence. They simply stood out too much. Under ordinary circumstances, few if any of them would present as transgender in a health care setting to protect themselves from violence. Yet the protocol required that they present themselves "normally" and in ways that did not hide their gender identification. As one of the Affirmative Action staff explained,

> A man in a man's clothing will have no problems until it is discovered he is a gay man. Then the doctor will start to discriminate against him. For a trans person, it is worse. Trans people are beaten up in the neighborhoods. One case happened just last week. They broke her legs they beat her so badly. Ask Gaston. He has photographs. We are far from achieving our objective.

Thea noted she risked "getting beat up" every time she went out to collect data, if she followed the protocol. There were also so few mystery patients that even with the high volume of patients these clinics managed, clinic staff might still come to recognize them over time. The fact of making repeat visits but not pursuing actual services might certainly also raise suspicion. Some worried they had already been found out. After the first mystery patient training, the mystery patients had trained their colleagues in turn, following local restitution practices, preparing others in their association to fulfill the role. Deploying these extra people as mystery patients might have allayed the concern of being discovered simply by creating a larger army of observers. But there was no money to support transportation costs for these additional observers.

The mystery patient role was also challenging to fulfill in part because a mystery patient must intentionally and repeatedly expose oneself to unpleasant, dangerous situations. Being a mystery patient puts one in the way of physical and psychological harm. Mystery patients reported they were denied entry to facilities and upbraided by security guards. Some reported they were sent away by nurses because their presence in the waiting rooms made other patients uncomfortable. Some were badgered as to whether they were male or female, as if their initial response did not suffice. Some were treated as if they were not standing in a queue or sitting in the waiting room at all; staff behaved as if they were not there. Some were openly mocked by staff. Unsurprisingly, mystery patients experienced these visits as stressful. They had experiences that generated intense anger and fear. The leaders who supervised the youngest of the mystery patients expressed concern about the mental health consequences for the young adults doing the work, concerns the mystery patients themselves echoed.[12] One association leader faulted the local project's design: "It wasn't easy to cope with the stress, so we organized a therapeutic group here. We had to seek solutions at the level of our own organization." Repeated exposure to degrading treatment without a formal mechanism to offer psychological support seemed to him like a major oversight. I agreed. I worried about their vulnerability to violence and of the consequences of the work on their mental health.

I shared a verbal summary of my findings from this visit with Johnny and with Guy before I left Cameroon. I followed up with them in writing once I had returned home. Guy and Johnny quickly began to brainstorm alternative procedures and identify ways to rebudget to put more resources toward safety. Guy brainstormed with Emil and Richard in parallel. As a first step, Affirmative Action established a mechanism for involving the identity organizations and mystery patients in devising revised procedures. They convened three listening sessions with mystery patients and leaders, three organizations at each. Coming together to share their experiences collecting data proved a transformative experience for the mystery patients. The staff of the nine organizations and of Affirmative Action strategized together around the mystery patients' concerns. In consultation with Positive Generation, they changed their data collection procedures to permit mystery patients to penetrate more deeply into each of the clinics. Thea described the listening session she participated in this way:

> At the phase 2 meeting, we had to take stock. That provided an opportunity to redirect the project. We talked about what challenges we were experiencing. We talked about our fears. We talked about the fact we were not at war. The phase 2 taking stock meeting helped us rethink the approach. We thought about our personal interests. We thought about what we wanted when the project ended. And that was motivation.

Another organizational leader commented, "It felt like at the check-up meetings they really tried to bring solutions." The country lead agreed: "The positive thing was their ability or their motivations to reflect and pivot." These sessions were significant for Affirmative Action, too, as they realized the benefits of an inclusive planning process. Reflecting on this experience, Emil later observed, "MPact taught us to focus on impact in every action that we take. To keep our eyes on the beneficiaries."

Following the listening sessions, Affirmative Action deployed all the trained mystery patients, whether they were originally trained by Positive Generation or via a restitution training, ensuring that if a mystery patient required a break from the stresses of data collection, they could take it. In consultation with the MPact country lead, Affirmative Action moved funds to cover the fees for initial medical consultations and for safe transportation to and from the clinics. Mystery patients could now seek screening for sexually transmitted infections or a basic medical consultation. For Thea, the meetings to plot a change of course proved vital to her sense of the project's importance and the importance of her role. She realized, she told me, she was doing this work for the whole community:

> You need the data. You must be informed. You must think of others. If we know what the stakes are, we know our ordinary purpose. We must think about those who are relying on us for the data that we are to collect. At the coordination meeting, we discussed this. We talked about what it meant to be a mystery patient. In the second phase, we had the support to go further.

Conclusion

The Project ACT partners' resilience resided in their rapid and agile response to problems and openness to learning. The resources guiding partners through moments of adversity and challenge were seldom if ever monetary. Rather, they were principally interpersonal and intrapersonal. Most of the Project ACT partners appear to take immense joy in their work. All are deeply committed to it. They readily work despite financial strain and risks to their personal security. A spirit of camaraderie and shared vision buoyed these teams through their roughest patches and over the obstacles created by a rushed and incomplete planning process. From the fire in Jamaica to the new strategies for mystery patient deployment and support in Cameroon, the partners benefited from their relationships to others, from incorporating deliberative, reflective, and inclusive approaches to navigating through challenges, and from leaders who viewed adversity as a learning opportunity. Finally, the spread-betting strategy in which collateral pathways were followed to achieve a singular goal saved the day not just in Jamaica. It also proved itself key to how a small demonstration project like Project ACT could accomplish as much as it did with only a little bit of money and a little bit of time.

8
With a Little Bit of Money and a Little Bit of Time

Laurent slowly cruised down the nondescript residential street in the heart of Quartier Gobele, skillfully avoiding the ruts carved into the roadbed's red soil. He idled for a moment alongside a metal compound door in the middle of the block, checking its description against the instructions he had stored in his phone. He cut the engine and then used WhatsApp to alert me that he was waiting outside. I grabbed my backpack off the cool stone tile floor, exited from the salon, and stepped outdoors into a furnace's blast of humid tropical morning air. I nodded to the gardener, who was crouching alongside a garden path, and to the security guard seated nearby. I opened the gate leading to the street where Laurent sat in his steel blue Mercedes, a stately relic of the early 1980s. The guard silently pulled the gate shut behind me.

"Bonjour, Laurent. Ça va bien?" I queried through the open car window, as Laurent toyed with his phone.

"You're practicing," he responded. "I am fine by God's grace, Madame Miller."

I climbed into the passenger seat. As I positioned my backpack between my legs, Laurent turned the key in the ignition. The car trembled slightly. Laurent popped the clutch. The car lurched and stalled out. He started the car again. It rumbled to life once more. Laurent smoothly engaged first gear. We headed through the streets of Abidjan's second plateau, windows open wide to the day's blistering heat, radio on. We stopped briefly so I could purchase a day's worth of diesel. With just over a quarter tank now in her belly, Laurent piloted the old Mercedes northwest to pick up the A1 toward Abobo.

Laurent is one of two community members who aided me as a translator during my visits to Côte d'Ivoire. He and I spent that day in early February 2020 touring radio stations in the northern suburbs of Abidjan and interviewing two of the radio journalists who had participated in Project ACT. Two days later, we traveled to Mermoz for a radio station tour and interview with a third journalist. In combination, over the course of 2019, the three journalists had broadcast 23 radio programs focused on the constitutional right of LGBT people to have access to health care free from stigma, discrimination, and violence. The journalists did so after having attended training provided to them by Claude and the staff of REPMASCI (Chapter 6), training intended to improve their understanding of the role journalists might play in providing Ivoirian citizens with sound information about HIV and sexual and gender minority people. Each of the journalists told me that the training they had received and the

Breaking Barriers. Robin Lin Miller and George Ayala, Oxford University Press. © Oxford University Press 2024.
DOI: 10.1093/oso/9780197647684.003.0009

connections that they formed to the representatives from community-led organizations who had also participated in the training sessions enabled them to make the programs they aired. Without the training, they said, they would not have had the tools or connections necessary to develop programs they believed were compelling, informative, sensitizing, and accurate in their depiction of LGBT people and their health concerns. The training solidified their commitment to produce sound journalism on the issues. It changed the language they use on air, too. They ceased using the derogatory and dehumanizing slang that was once part of their ordinary on-air vocabulary: "I used to refer to gay men as 'PD.' Now I know the good terminology," one shared.[1] Another commented, "The knowledge I gained has changed the words I use."

Each of the three journalists successfully pushed their very reluctant station managers to allow them to create and air these rare programs. They broadcasted on topics including transgender people, gay and bisexual men, lesbian and bisexual women, the constitutional rights of LGBT people to health and well-being, safety when accessing health care, and the vital role of community-led organizations in addressing the HIV epidemic. The programs featured LGBT people speaking for themselves about themselves. The LGBT community members who went on the air were typically affiliated with one of the three community-led organizations—Arc en Ciel, QET Inclusion, and Secours Social—that had participated in the training with the journalists and who were themselves trained through Project ACT in making small media videos.

The journalists aired several live broadcasts during which listeners could call in. On his first live broadcast, the journalist from Abobo featured two gay male guests. Reflecting on that program, he observed, "1 hour was not enough. We got many more calls than normal." I asked about the nature of those calls. He told me callers often expressed negative views in response to the program, but that it also generated supportive comments. "The feedback was mixed, with some saying, 'We are all brothers and sisters,' and 'People should be allowed to live their lives, as long as they stay away from children,' and others saying it was not natural." The journalist broadcasting from the station in Anyama reported that he had received similar caller reactions to his first live program. "Three out of five callers said things like 'We have to kill them.' The rest said, 'It is their life, and we should leave them alone.'"

Station managers function as the gatekeepers of the content journalists can share with the public. The fact that the first live programs aired by the journalists generated above-average numbers of audience calls helped the journalists to convince their station managers to air more programs. "I made one show as an audition," the Abobo journalist said, referring to his first live program "and, was finally permitted to produce three on gay men. The first received enough calls that management accepted me doing two more." Building on his initial success, he invited a physician and representatives of a human rights advocacy organization to come on air. Next, he aired a program on bisexuality and then one in which he invited religious leaders to talk about the issues facing "key populations." "Live programs bringing on gay people and straight people to confront one another was not possible to do before," he said. The journalist broadcasting out of Anyama reported a similar experience. "My media director is a woman who did not agree to our airing these programs," he told me immediately before introducing me to her. When we were alone again, he offered that she is a pious woman who holds strong negative views on homosexuality. At first, he explained, she was only willing to permit him to air programs that focused on health care. Nothing else. What is more, she told him that he alone had to bear all responsibility for the programs. She only permitted him to continue broadcasting shows on LGBT health and HIV because of the high volume of call-in responses the broadcasts generated. Although he endured the scorn of colleagues at the station, he pressed on. Little by little, he expanded the content of his reporting.

Airing these radio programs proved challenging not only because of the initial reticence of station managers to permit the content on the airwaves that they control. The representatives from the community-led organizations, while enthusiastic about working with the media during the safety of the training sessions, were overcome by fear when their time to go on the radio arrived. "They were afraid. On a live program, they were afraid someone was waiting outside." The Anyama journalist quickly learned that if he wanted to bring these programs to his listeners, he had to develop safety measures to protect his guests. "I ensured their safety while in the district. I escorted them to and from the station. I do use consents," he said pointing to the evaluation consent document laying on the table in the broadcasting booth where he and I sat, "but I don't take photos or videos of people." He decided to prerecord about 60% of his programs to allay guests' fears and to assure them he could protect their safety. The Abobo journalist expressed similar caution about doing live programs. The journalist in Mermoz opted for prerecorded programs, too, although he hoped to do live programming in the future. Each believed in the value of live programs but recognized the validity of community members' hesitation. "The community stigma is so high they were not ready to participate when called. Journalists need them in order to do the work," one lamented.

Airing radio programs on the barriers to accessing health care for gay and bisexual men and transgender women on radio stations in Côte d'Ivoire is a signature achievement of the local work performed by Alternative Côte d'Ivoire and REPMASCI. Media directors and station managers are profit driven. According to Claude, they cannot air programs that will not "sell," which drives them to focus on national events, murders, and sensationalized content. "It is normal to refuse to do things on gay people except on World AIDS Day," he added. Regularly airing balanced, scientifically informed programs that portray sexual and gender minority people as human beings who are entitled to equal rights reflected a tremendous narrative shift from the typical radio broadcast. Putting LGBT people on air as part of that programming permitted the community to shape its own narrative, raise its visibility, and normalize their health concerns. People were listening to these programs. They called in. They engaged in public debate.

The behavioral changes reflected in this achievement—station managers consenting to air novel content, journalists creating innovative programming and adopting neutral on-air language, community members appearing on the air to share their experiences and perspectives—are the types of observable changes in the behavior of people and institutions that an outcome-harvesting approach (Wilson-Grau, 2018; Wilson-Grau & Britt, 2012) is designed to detect: a novel behavior that is readily verifiable, of clear local significance, and for which the contribution of a policy or project is logical and traceable. Outcomes are meaningful in context; they contribute to moving in a desired direction. In Côte d'Ivoire, attention to sexual and gender minority issues in mainstream media is unusual. The kind of reporting resulting from the activities of Project ACT may contribute to a change in public perceptions of sexual and gender minority people toward greater tolerance. This is the kind of media reporting that has the potential to enhance rights-based access to HIV care.

These are not the only outcomes I observed in Côte d'Ivoire, nor was this the only instance in which a Project ACT partner contributed to shifting public narratives by securing mainstream press reportage. But Alternative Côte d'Ivoire was the only partner that hoped to influence the media. During the end-of-project workshop that we held in Rwanda to take stock of the project and identify what we had learned, the Project ACT partners completed an adapted exercise based on most-significant-change storytelling (Davies & Dart, 2005). Each partner composed two most-significant-change stories. This story—journalists airing unbiased programs on diverse topics of vital importance to the local LGBT community—was voted the most significant change of all by the Project ACT partners. Portraying their communities in positive and relatable ways on multiple radio stations was as unfamiliar to partners as it was a stunning success.

Building and Setting New Agendas

The successes the Ivorians experienced fell short of their own hopes but provide a clear example of how Project ACT enabled its partners to build on the foundations of their past work to shift the ways in which relevant issues were covered, framed, and delivered; ensure that evidence was used in support of desired messages; and engage new actors in delivering messages. In addition to putting novel radio content on the air, Alternative Côte d'Ivoire succeeded in bringing Secours Social's short videos to the attention of a national mainstream human rights organization. That organization now uses these videos to bring national attention to LGBT issues and human rights violations committed against sexual and gender minority people. Claude claimed the training sessions had inspired a journalist to conceive a book.[2] Despite the fits, starts, and tensions in their relationship (Chapter 6), Alternative Côte d'Ivoire and REPMASCI stimulated increased attention to LGBT issues in mainstream media outlets, including print resources. Alternative Côte d'Ivoire and REPMASCI helped set a new agenda for public discourse, elevating the importance of rights-based access to health care in the public's eye.

Agenda building and setting occurred in other Project ACT countries, including Burundi, Cameroon, Jamaica, and Zimbabwe. In Burundi, the project focused heavily on mobilizing community-led groups to gain access to the policy processes that impact on HIV health services. LBGT communities participated in formulating recommendations for the PEPFAR Country Operational Plan planning process for the first time, improving the odds that the needs of the community were voiced and considered in the development of Burundi's 2021 plan. Indeed, novel elements in the 2021 plan include the intention to shift oversight of the "key populations" program that focuses on gay, bisexual, and other men who have sex with men from the government to a "KP competent" organization that subcontracts with community-led organizations. The plan also supports structural intervention programming to decrease stigma, discrimination, and violence (PEPFAR, 2021).

In Cameroon, during my final audience with the Secretary General of the National Commission on Human Rights and Freedoms, she shared that she was actively applying what she learned from the project's sensitization trainings and from closely observing the project's implementation into the national 5-year action plan for the HIV/TB human rights framework. The training helped her think about how to create feasible and impactful strategies that recognize the importance of all hospital jobs in promoting human rights and dignity. Her integration of lessons from Project ACT's implementation into a national framework allows messages on the importance of affirming health care to reach all levels of Cameroon's health care ecosystem.

After brainstorming with her country lead on how to embed advocacy messages into the national Transgender Health and Wellness Conference that she organized, Dymond developed a call to action. The call demanded the Jamaican government systematically collect data on transgender people and their experiences to improve the quality of health care in Jamaica. The call to action was featured in an article that appeared in a national newspaper on July 1, 2019 (*Jamaica Observer*), creating the potential to build public support for the rights of transgender people to health care. The Jamaican National Family Planning Board followed up on the call by establishing a partnership with TransWave to work on the issues that Dymond had identified. A policy brief the J-FLAG team authored provided the ethical argument and evidentiary support for a motion that was introduced into Parliament on decriminalizing abortion. The abortion statute appears in the Jamaican Offences Against the Person Act, which also criminalizes same-sex sexual relationships. The motion, which drew multiple supporters, prompted national discussion on individual rights to health care and on human rights regarding privacy and bodily autonomy. Leveraging the overlap of gendered forms of oppression in its development of the brief (Chapter 6), J-FLAG's advocates gained a seat at the policymaking table, actively informing the discussion held among Members of Parliament and cementing a new ally in Parliament in the process. The Jamaican team also capitalized on its bridge-building conversations (Chapter 6), cementing a partnership with the British Health Commission to address employment discrimination.

In Zimbabwe, the 10 peer mobilizers met regularly throughout the project to brainstorm ideas for supplementary efforts they could pursue to educate others about HIV, sensitize people regarding LGBT issues, and advocate for broad social change. For instance, they initiated a four-part series of sexuality dialogues on a local college campus. They successfully developed abstracts about their work and presented them at the 2019 International Conference on AIDS and STIs in Africa (ICASA). One of the mobilizers, Blessing, spoke on a panel concerning legal barriers to HIV services for young people. I, Robin, sat in the audience with Zandi, Mandla, another peer mobilizer, Siphosenkosi, and the other Sexual Rights Centre staff who attended the conference to hear Blessing speak. The audience was full. Blessing led off the youth on the panel, speaking eloquently about the issues facing young gay and bisexual men in Zimbabwe and the role law played in creating a disabling environment for their accessing sexual and reproductive health care services. As it happened, three parliamentarians also attended his session, two from Uganda and one from Sierra Leone. During the question-and-answer part of the session, the policymaker from Sierra Leone sought Blessing's advice on how to improve his country's environment for youth like himself. One of the Ugandan officials quickly followed in turn. Both officials sought him out after the session. The Ugandan parliamentarian requested Blessing's ongoing consultation on how to ensure the safety of LGBT delegates to ICASA 2021, which Uganda was scheduled to host.[3] When I asked Blessing later if he continued his interactions with the two dignitaries, he indicated that he had follow-up conversations with the Ugandan parliamentarian. This last example of how Project ACT's local activities contributed to agenda setting illustrates the value of the empowering settings the Sexual Rights Centre created for its young peer mobilizers (Chapter 5). Empowering settings can build young men's confidence about sharing their experiences publicly. Empowering young gay and bisexual men to share their expertise and insights, as the peer mobilizers did in their poster session and Blessing did on the stage that day, may inspire similar efforts elsewhere in Zimbabwe and in other African countries. Young men's exposure to and increased visibility within forums like ICASA 2019—which includes a sizeable political delegation of heads of state and their spouses, parliamentarians, and government officials—may inspire other young men to engage with the HIV epidemic in new ways. It can create novel opportunities for them. Attracting the attention of high-level duty bearers and evolving relationships with them can ensure that politicians attune to the challenges faced by the LGBT community in accessing health care.

Altering Norms and Eliminating Exclusionary Practices

The advocacy work performed by the Project ACT partners contributed to shifts in the discretionary norms and practices that maintain inequitable access to and poor treatment in health care settings. In Cameroon, the three largest HIV outpatient treatment facilities in Yaoundé's Nkolodongo, Biyem-Assi, and Cité Verte health districts were the targets of mystery patient data collection: the day clinics of Central and Biyem-Assi District hospitals, and a clinic operated by the Cameroon National Association for Family Welfare, an affiliate of the International Planned Parenthood Federation. Each of these clinics has high patient volumes of people living with HIV, with the highest, Central Hospital, peaking at about 10,000 people living with HIV per year, according to the chief physician. Affirmative Action and their partner, Positive Generation (Chapter 6), designed a sensitization training informed by the mystery patient data they were collecting and with guidance provided to them by their MPact country lead.[4] They delivered the initial training session as a 5-day retreat for 30 people—the leaders of the targeted outpatient facilities, the heads of the health districts in which the facilities were located, select staff from each facility, and a small number of high-ranking government officials—in Douala. Afterward, Affirmative Action held a training session in each district for health care workers and district leadership. Following the local norm of restitution, the district heads and five of the health care workers who had attended the Douala retreat, co-led these training sessions. All the training sessions culminated in the development of 2-year facility- and district-level action plans for change.

The trainings opened with a discussion of the data obtained from two rounds of mystery patient data collection[5] and the testimonials of two mystery patients, one a young gay man and the second a transgender woman (Thea). The combination of highly detailed quantitative data on stigma and discrimination, coupled with testimonial descriptions of experiences in the facilities, shook trainees. One of the reference physicians from Central Hospital's clinic later reflected, "We have a better understanding of what it takes for them to go to a doctor's office. The testimonials stood out. The naming of the hospitals. That was the powerful part." The quantitative data embarrassed and concerned the health care workers, but it was the testimony provided by Thea that moved them most. Almost every person—the district heads, physicians, nurses, and other health care workers I interviewed in March of 2020—recounted pieces of Thea's testimony. In one interview, my translator (Chantal), two physicians, a nurse, and I crowded into a small narrow room, the windows and doors open to the sounds of the teeming hospital campus and echoes of the crowded patient corridor. One of the physicians recounted parts of the training that I would hear recounted multiple times by others:

> She [Thea] told a story of being in a hospital waiting room seated between two pregnant women. The women shifted away from her. They whispered to one another, moving, fearful their unborn child might catch the same disease. They preferred to stand. She told another story of being laughed at by a nurse who, after seeing her, went to get her coworkers from the back to come out. They stood in the doorway and stared and laughed. Thea had to call on all her strength to stay there in the face of repugnant treatment.

Thea's stories prompted the physician to ask herself what she could do to improve access to care. The other physician participating in our conversation concluded it by stating, "They have been made to be sick because of stigma and discrimination," a realization she carried with her months later.

Discovering that other patients in the waiting rooms behaved in a stigmatizing manner was among the insights from that training that prompted swift change. The day clinic at Central Hospital revised its patient orientation counseling to include human rights education. The new orientation addresses the human right of all Cameroonians to seek care in the clinic. It discourages patients from stigmatizing others seeking care. Physicians and nurses developed procedures to permit their sexual and gender minority patients to experience minimal wait times or avoid the waiting room all together, recognizing it might not be entirely possible to guarantee a stigma-free waiting room. Community members now call their providers' cell phones when they arrive on site.[6] The district heads and facility leaders developed a 2-year action plan to improve the welcoming process for patients. The district heads and clinic leaders noted that during the training, they came to realize a whole-facility approach was necessary. Encountering poor treatment in any unit of the hospital or when seeking any service might discourage sexual and gender minority people from pursuing HIV care. Although the process will be slow, given the size of the facilities, Central Hospital's leaders stated the intent to provide sensitization training to all its 700 employees, right down to the security guards. Central Hospital was not anomalous in its efforts. By the time the project concluded, the Biyem-Assi District Hospital had begun to implement a new client feedback system, had hung signage throughout its day clinic facility indicating that stigma and discrimination have no place in health care, and had created a new system of supervision and provider monitoring to assess the quality of treatment being received by sexual and gender minority patients. Remaking the physical environment, including affirming signage, also occurred in Zimbabwe and Ghana.

In Ghana and Zimbabwe, the use of mystery patients to capture stigma and discrimination and develop redress systems, although implemented differently than in Cameroon (Chapter 5), also led to similar changes in health care workers' and administrators' behavior. In Ghana, a redress system evolved out of empowerment training and the use of mystery patients to identify affirming facilities throughout the greater Accra region. When community members and mystery patients encountered problematic treatment, they made detailed reports to patient advocates at our partner organization. These reports led to sanctions against health care employees. A pharmacist was investigated for having disclosed private patient information to a patient's friend. After the allegation that he had shared privileged health information was proven true, he lost his position. Nurses were disciplined for divulging private patient information to an adult patient's mother without his prior knowledge or consent. Nurses were also investigated for engaging in discriminatory behavior. In Zimbabwe, the new mystery patient and redress system also led to individual-level performance feedback. Not all responded favorably to these new systems. In Zimbabwe, some health care employees complained that the new system led to false and unfair accusations and to undue privileged treatment of young gay and bisexual men. In other countries, health care workers reported they now shouldered the stigma and rejection of their colleagues for their attempts at change. However, dialogue among health care leaders, providers, and community members about what constituted a stigma-free encounter and patient rights was becoming institutionalized, as was the emergence of cooperative relationships among provider institutions, community activists, and sexual and gender minority constituents.

As we have already shown, notable shifts in political consciousness and commitment grew out of efforts at sensitization. In Cameroon, after the Douala sensitization training, the health district heads from Nkoldongo, Biyem-assi, and Cité Verte formed their own WhatsApp group to keep in communication with one another about contemporary and emerging issues affecting gay and bisexual men and transgender women. They used the group to stay in routine contact with LGBT community-led organizations. They also started to use each other as a sounding board for making progress toward opening access to care in their districts' facilities. The medical directors from two of the three main prisons in Yaoundé attended the Doula training. They voluntarily requested special follow-up training for their entire prison health care staff from Affirmative Action, an extraordinary step given these prisons' notoriety. Their poor treatment of sexual and gender minority people who have been incarcerated in these facilities on supposed violation of Cameroon's criminalization code is widely known.[7]

Improving Access to Health Care Resources

Although many of these changes represent steps toward structural improvements in access, they may seem to some readers to fall short of improving access to health care resources. Remarkably, over the short duration of the project, concrete improvements in access also occurred. In several of the countries, sensitization training and the direct interactions these trainings fostered between community members and health care providers led health care providers to recognize that stigmatized populations may prefer to pursue care in settings that they already perceive as safe and affirming. Providers initiated the establishment of new on-site service offerings at community-led organizations. A physician reached out to a well-regarded Cameroonian community-led organization with a large constituency of people living with HIV to establish on-site clinical services. Two other physicians and a mental health specialist did the same, ensuring consistent health care services at this location. In Zimbabwe, the local Population Services International clinic (PSI), one of the two health care facilities that the project targeted, opened a Wednesday morning clinic at the Sexual Rights Centre's headquarters, a space already perceived as safe and that attracts large numbers of young gay and bisexual men. One benefit of these latter arrangements, besides improving access to basic HIV services in community-led settings, is the boost in reputation that comes from direct outreach. The clinics in which these providers work quickly became known as resources that offer sensitive HIV care, after having demonstrated their commitment to the LGBT population through their partnership with community-led groups. Referral patterns shifted to institutions and individual providers cooperating with Project ACT and to those affirmed as delivering respectful and sensitive care through mystery patient documentation. In Ghana, through mystery patient documentation, our partner affirmed 20 clinics in the greater Accra region provided stigma-free care. Our partner now publicizes these clinics to the community as facilities with verified stigma-free practices. In Zimbabwe, gay and bisexual men now receive referrals to the health care workers who have at least a minimum preparation for responding to their health concerns with sensitivity and who have made a commitment to fair service provision. Trained providers, and those who come on site to offer care, typically gain these referrals.

Insights gained from mystery patients led to additional changes in referral patterns. The realizations that mystery patients themselves gained altered access to resources in unexpected ways. Mystery patients in Cameroon discovered that their experiences at the facility with the best reputation in the LGBT community were often poor compared with their expectations. Similarly, they found their experiences at a facility with a poor reputation were far better than they expected, at least among the cisgender mystery patients. Two organizations changed their referrals to the places where the data collected by their constituents indicated the fewest negative and most frequent positive experiences. One of the organizations went further. They chose to seek an alternative referral source, one that was not part of the mystery patient investigations. That decision led to a formal relationship with a private hospital and to the hospital offering on-site nursing services at the community-led organization's headquarters.

The importance of these gains in access to care may appear modest at first. But gay and bisexual men and transgender women are more likely to accept and remain engaged in services when they interact with health care workers who treat them with compassion and an absence of bias (Ayala et al., 2022; Ayala & Santos, 2016). When health care workers gain the reputation as affirming providers, this creates a reinforcing system. As gay and bisexual men's and transgender women's confidence in certain providers grows, word of mouth spreads that the community can expect to be well cared for by these providers. In turn, the numbers of gay and bisexual men and transgender women who are HIV tested and linked to biomedical prevention and treatment may increase. Improved access to HIV care means that more gay and bisexual men and transgender women will know their HIV status and receive pre-exposure prophylaxis (PrEP), condoms, lubricant, antiretroviral therapy, and sexually transmitted infection treatment.

Formal Policies

Changes to formal rules laid down in policy or the allocation of financial and other resources, although rare, occurred. The PSI clinic in Zimbabwe adopted a policy that all new employees, regardless of their role, undergo sensitization training as part of their onboarding process. The government hospital, Mpilo, entered a formal Memorandum of Understanding with the Sexual Rights Centre. The most sweeping policy change occurred in República Dominicana. Despite Project ACT's slow start there, it secured a shining achievement: the Dominican Ministry of Health entered a two-party Memorandum of Understanding with Amigos Siempre Amigos that guarantees health care workers' attendance at two-day sensitization workshops. The government took responsibility for issuing the call to training and established a national training calendar, ensuring sensitization is a standard practice and a national priority for effective service provision. This government partnership, and the one in Zimbabwe, are especially significant because community-led organizations initiated these partnerships.

Enhanced Advocacy Capacity

Every positive step we have described (and others we have not described here) came about through growth in the skills, relationships, resources, and will on which advocacy initiatives such as this depend. Blessing and his peers' development as advocates provide a clear example of building the local advocacy capacity necessary to sustain human rights movements and the success such efforts yield. These 10 young men enhanced their skills in advocacy through a solid foundation of training and through executing the core work of mobilizing other young men to use health care, thereby normalizing the presence of young gay and bisexual men in local health care systems. These activities produced cascading benefits in growing the local capacity for advocacy. The peer mobilizers' training and project experiences reinvigorated the two Sexual Rights Centre collectives devoted to young gay and bisexual men. Their memberships expanded. Their missions enlarged. The peer mobilizers provided testimony of their experiences to decision makers from Zimbabwe's Parliamentary Portfolio on Health and Gender, and to representatives of the National AIDS Control Committee, UNAIDS, and the United Nations Population Fund (UNFPA). Engaging with these multilateral organizations, Parliamentarians, officials, and country-level leaders paves the way for creating a more enabling policy environment. But it also represents progress toward realizing two of the pillars of a human rights advocacy framework: holding duty-bearers to account and civic participation of rights holders.

The mystery patients of Cameroon provide another example of expanded advocacy skills. Drawing on their newfound skills in data collection, a group of mystery patients created a systematic observational methodology to conduct a community-led environmental risk assessment of high-risk hotspots for LGBT violence. The map of Yaoundé they produced provides the LGBT community a safety guide and a tool for advocating with local police to better protect the community. Transgender people in Jamaica learned to write letters to the editor and to speak in public fora. Impressively, Dymond and her colleagues prepared the first-ever transgender-specific submission on transgender rights for Jamaica's Universal Periodic Review.[8] The growth in TransWave, and in Dymond as its leader, is notable. Dymond credits Project ACT with building her capacity and increasing the capacity for transgender activism in Jamaica. "I started as the only employee when you first came," she told me. "Now we are up to 6 or 7. We owe that to MPact." Project ACT and her relationship to MPact created other valuable opportunities for her, including participation in a transnational training program on increasing demand for PrEP and seed money to start a PrEP-demand program in Jamaica.

Developing a public base of support for a movement and encouraging the development of those who are willing to engage in a movement are part of building the people power necessary for change to occur. The journalists of Côte d'Ivoire and their efforts to use media platforms to win public support of LGBT rights to access health care are exemplars of the expanded person power to which Project ACT contributed. As part of the work in Zimbabwe, MPact's country lead provided an in-depth training to 10 health care workers who were willing to become champions in their work settings (Chapter 6). These health care workers strategized on two fronts: how they could have more influence on hospital management policies and practices, and how they could influence the nursing curriculum at Mpilo hospital to incorporate LGBT sensitization. The last time I met with them, the group was developing a plan to expose student nurses to introductory material on human sexuality. They were also positioning themselves to leverage external pressure on the hospital due to newfound national attention given to the role of stigma and discrimination as barriers to care. Just as the internal pressure individual journalists placed on their station managers led to novel broadcasts, internal pressure originating from inside a health care institution can enhance the likelihood of change to health care policy and practice. Inspired by this original cadre of health care champions, other health care workers requested training to become champions. Requests to become part of the project suggest it stimulated health care workers' desire to become stewards of the process to reduce stigma and discrimination. It stoked their willingness to take responsibility for ensuring gay and bisexual men and transgender women are well-served by the health care system. Expanding the number of health care workers who are willing to champion the needs and rights of gay and bisexual men and transgender women can only further ongoing changes in norms and attitudes at facilities like Mpilo and PSI. Nurse champions like those mobilized in Zimbabwe also emerged in other countries, notably Ghana. Nurses there routinely organized and offered training for their peers, developed improved patient scheduling and follow-up systems, and initiated other innovations to ensure provision of affirming care.

At the start of the project in Cameroon, Affirmative Action developed a short video outlining their project plans. They held a small, invitational launch event at which they showed the video. Upon seeing the video, the Permanent Secretary of the National AIDS Control Committee approached Guy. He requested that every certificate of completion from the sensitization training bear his signature. The Secretary General of the Commission on Human Rights and Freedoms, already an ally to the project, also lent her signature to these certificates. Each of the original mystery patients received a signed certificate at the end of the project. Each community-led organization and each targeted hospital received a framed certificate of excellence, approximately 20" × 24", signed by these high-ranking officials. These two officials publicly threw their weight behind the project in a first-of-its-kind partnership between government actors and LGBT-led community organizations, openly acknowledging the need to break down barriers to HIV care for gay and bisexual men and transgender women.

On my final day in Cameroon, Richard traveled across Yaoundé to present certificates to staff from two of the medical facilities and to eight of the community-led organizations and their mystery patients. Chantal and I accompanied him. We made our way gingerly down steep and rutted alleyways, some impassible to our truck. We climbed narrow concrete staircases floors up. One wound so tightly up a four-story spiral, its concrete crumbling, Chantal could not manage it in the heels she had selected to wear that day. Down these alleys and up these stairs, we passed through unmarked gates and entered unmarked doorways, toting the oversized gold-framed certificates of excellence and certificates of recognition. The Secretary General joined us at our first stop: the Cameroonian Association for AIDS (CAMFAIDS), the organization that Eric Lembebe led in 2013 when he was brutally murdered (Chapter 1). There, she presented certificates to the organization's leaders and to mystery patients. The significance of receiving a certificate bearing the signatures of high-ranking government officials was not lost to anyone who received one. The pictures Richard and I took to document the day reveal this, especially those we took of the mystery patients and the staff members of the community-led organizations. Holding their "Attestation de Bonne Execution," they beam at our cameras, overcome with delight and pride.

As every example of change we provide underscores, strengthened relationships to others increased local advocacy capacity. The Sexual Rights Centre strengthened its ties to GALZ, the oldest community-led organization in Zimbabwe, by inviting them to help build the skills of the second set of health care worker champions. They strengthened their ties to two major health care facilities by formalizing those relationships, something they would never have imagined as possible before. The government-run city clinic health system requested to join Project ACT. Our partner in Burundi created a formal national network out of a once loose confederation of community-led groups, establishing the potential for coordinated national documentation of and responses to human rights violations. Positive Generation and Affirmative Action, recognizing that they have greater influence by working together, continued their partnership. In these and other instances, Project ACT helped establish or enhance action-focused advocacy relationships.

Not every consequence of Project ACT reflects a desirable achievement. There are hopes that the partners did not realize. Everyone made missteps. But on December 9, 2019, when the Project ACT partners, the MPact team, and I gathered at the Onomo Hotel, overlooking the hills of Kimihurura, to take stock of what had occurred since we had gathered in Cambodia, we were all taken by surprise at what had been accomplished. Affirmative Action, Positive Generation, and their nine community-led organization partners had their toes in what once was a closed door, making it possible to create the system of loving care they had long hoped might come about in Yaoundé and creating a model for what they might do to open similar doors in other regions. For the first time, they had a formal, cooperative partnership with the highest levels of government. J-FLAG had cemented new relationships in Parliament and with key influencers in the business, education, and other social sectors. They had promoted the growth and development of Jamaica's first transgender community-led advocacy organization, leading to a national call for action on transgender health and rights and a UPR submission on transgender concerns. Amigos Siempre Amigos had secured the government's commitment for guaranteed attendance of health care workers at sensitization trainings to promote affirming care to sexual and gender minority people. Our Ghanaian partner had documented and reported human rights abuses in health care. They established stigma-free zones and community-certified stigma-free facilities throughout greater Accra. Alternative Côte d'Ivoire had put LGBT issues in the public's eye through videos, radio broadcasts, and community-made videos. The Burundians had created and trained a coordinated network of nascent community-led organizations across five provinces and provided them with tools to document human rights violations. They had secured a voice at the planning table for the COP. The Sexual Rights Centre, through its quarterly review of mystery patient data, sensitization, and internal advocacy champions, had helped remake PSI as a center of excellence and Mpilo as an emerging center of excellence. The city clinics wanted in. These are breathtaking achievements over just 18 months. They demonstrate what activists can do with just a little bit of money and time when granted the flexibility to apply their expertise. As the journalist from Mermoz told me, as I stood to leave his radio station, "It was good, but very short."

9
There Will Be No Protests Here

We began the story of Project ACT by situating sexual and gender minority community-led organizations operating in parts of the Global South within their daily practical realities[1]. These realities include working in country contexts in which the daily tasks of outreach, engagement, and community building; of educating about sexual and gender minority people and their health concerns; and of linking people to HIV testing and care increases the odds of enduring harassment, violence, blackmail, arrest, and other forms of abuse. Realities in which institutions founded to champion sexual and gender minority people's rights and needs encounter undue barriers to their legal recognition as legitimate institutions, find their public voice policed, and guard their visibility by necessity of their security. Realities in which financial support of their efforts is principally owed to foreign donors, who often impose operating norms and programmatic objectives and indicators as conditions of their funding that are neither driven by nor in sync with community priorities and perspectives. Realities in which transnational intermediaries often unwittingly mirror their donors' prerogatives and adopt their assumptions about what is most beneficial. Realities in which the dominant perspective on sexual and gender minority people demonizes them and portrays them as subhuman deviants whose misdeeds warrant criminalization, rebuke, rejection, and correction.[2] Realities in which a visit to a doctor or nurse can be an exercise in enduring degradation and humiliation. Realities in which love, joy, pleasure, sex, and community are driven from public view and expression into secret spaces. Realities in which it is simply impossible to ignore these overwhelming dynamics of power and vulnerability to focus on the simplified version of the optimum HIV response promulgated by donors and governments. Realities in which ending AIDS requires far more than mere routine HIV test administration and medication distribution. What does HIV human rights advocacy led by local actors look like in these places?

The Practice and Contributions of Sexual and Gender Minority Community-Led Advocacy

A central purpose of this book is to explore how sexual and gender minority community-led organizations push forward an HIV agenda that acknowledges the dynamics of power and vulnerability in which their communities are enmeshed and begins the slow process of tearing down structural impediments to humane and

Breaking Barriers. Robin Lin Miller and George Ayala, Oxford University Press. © Oxford University Press 2024.
DOI: 10.1093/oso/9780197647684.003.0010

accessible HIV care. The story of Project ACT reveals a closely tied community of sexual and gender minority people (Chapters 3 and 4) and a handful of their allies (Chapter 6) strategically identifying and pursuing actions targeted directly at the people who sit at points of leverage in local systems of power. The targeted focus on a handful of journalists who proved willing to risk their reputations and jobs to produce sound journalism and establish their radio stations as pioneers, on influencers in ministries, health districts, and health care facilities with large enrollments of people living with HIV and a willingness to act on their belief in beneficent medical systems, and on parliamentarians committed to adjacent rights issues (Chapter 8) offered Project ACT partners toeholds in these systems through which they could stimulate internal movements for change. The cascading effect of these targeted advocacy initiatives, and the relationships formed on the edges of those cascades, were apparent in nearly every Project ACT setting. The outcomes we uncovered, however modest in the view of those who focus narrowly on end-game metrics, led to others and again to others. And with these outcomes, new relationships were born upon which additional advocacy opportunities, and in turn advocacy wins, would spring. This is the nature of advocacy led by sexual and gender minority people across Africa, the Caribbean, and, very possibly, the world. Nothing that happened in these places was perfect and neat in its planning and execution. Nonetheless, the tactics partners deployed succeeded in setting desirable changes in motion.

In every one of the Project ACT countries, the partners to Project ACT and their allies made steps toward creating an environment that enables access to HIV care and improves the likelihood of receiving affirming care. Despite the long odds of making steps toward change, Project ACT contributed to more than 100 verified outcomes[3] (and probably more, given limits to our evaluation resources and the interruption to our final data collection caused by COVID-19 travel lockdowns). The sheer number of wins evident over the brief timeframe of 18 months of active work in the field and despite persistent obstacles, historical events, and other challenges (Chapter 7) is noteworthy. Modest wins may not prove inconsequential in the longer run, a bet that is inherent to incremental pursuits like advocacy. No Project ACT partner held the delusion of sweeping overnight change. Instead, working from the ground up, they focused on what was immediate and local. They focused on the path to an enabling environment.

Some Project ACT sites went farther faster. Those that made the most visible and substantial progress did so working in close alliances and through the deployment of a multipronged, setting-specific strategy. The hostility of their context did not impede them noticeably once their partnerships were well cemented, however difficult some of these relationships proved to navigate (Chapter 6). Diversity in actions aided progress (Chapter 7). The combined strategies of deploying mystery patient documentation, coupled with sensitization practices, proved especially valuable in developing new champions of the community's cause and illustrates the benefits of adopting a multipronged approach. Documentation, through mystery patients, permitted change to occur along two distinct pathways. Along the first, when gay and bisexual men and transgender women found that they had consistently positive experiences in a health care setting, word of mouth spread "like a bush fire," as Gaston from Cameroon put it, increasing demand for services in those facilities and from the providers who offered affirming care. This process fed on itself. Documentation aided community members in exercising their power to select from available sources of care in an informed manner.

Along the second pathway, documentation permitted the community to hold up a mirror to health care providers and administrators. The image the community displayed often took those providers and administrators by surprise, prompting deep examination of their workplace practices and personal beliefs, and opening a community-provider dialogue on system reforms. One district leader in Cameroon offered her explanation of why documentation catapulted her into action: "I believe in evidence. Lack of evidence is not credible. Statistics mean that something is real. Statistics showed me that homosexuality really exists in Africa." She went on. "The data clearly showed patients experience stigma and discrimination and that they may not go to get care because of it." By providing credible documentation to health care providers and officials, this strategy united the community and its provider institutions in creating new systems of shared stewardship. By itself, what documentation accomplished struck every Project ACT partner who did not use this approach as worth adding to their advocacy portfolios.[4]

Sensitization practices were a powerful and complementary tool, but especially when sharing testimonial stories were included. Stories enlightened providers to the ordinary experiences of sexual and gender minority people. A growing body of evidence in social psychology indicates that intervention techniques, such as the use of testimonial stories, enhance perspective taking (Dovido et al., 2004; Paluck & Green, 2009; Todd & Galinsky, 2014). Perspective taking refers to the active consideration of another's mental state. Perspective-taking interventions increase empathetic responding and recognition of our similarities to others. Perspective taking also decreases the tendency to attribute others' suffering to their personal attributes rather than to their circumstances. Although perspective-taking interventions are understudied in field settings, emergent evidence from both the lab and the field suggests intervention approaches informed by perspective taking are promising for reducing prejudice (see, for example, Mousa, 2020; Simonovits et al., 2018).

The qualitative data we collected demonstrate that mystery patient testimonials stimulated the kinds of emotional and cognitive processes indicative of perspective taking. The same district head from Cameroon quoted earlier pointed to the testimonials as more impactful than statistics because, in her words, this is where she really understood that health care staff behave in ways that "punish, mock, and degrade people who are there to be cared for." Listeners met dimensional human beings in the particulars of testimonial stories. Through stories, providers came to recognize sexual and gender minority people as like the people in their own lives, people whom they treasured: spouses, children, siblings, parents, uncles, aunts, neighbors. They saw themselves, too, and their potential to harm. The sensitization methodology, as it was experienced, directly "spoke to the conscience" and forced an intimacy or closeness that complemented the abstraction of numbers. "It helped us to see these people are not wicked," one physician explained. "We see the cultural, religious and legal context molds us to see them that way." Another commented, "Being together for 5 days. Mingling. Eating. Nothing happened! That was normalizing." The sensitization component contributed to the development of empathy (Muwanguzi et al., 2023) and the formation of an emotional connection, while the covertly collected data catalyzed action (Daouk-Öyry et al., 2018) driven by aspirations for health care quality. Deployed in combination, we found these strategies resulted in concrete actions to ensure improved access to health care and enhanced engagement of health care professionals, community-led organizations, and sexual and gender minority constituents as partners in breaking down barriers. Praising this combination of strategies and their appropriateness to her country context, a physician observed "major changes resulting from major actions and protests, that will not happen here." These strategies worked well together, she told me, because they established closeness.

Principles of Practice

Through Project ACT, we divined principles of practice useful to guiding advocacy in our partners' country environments, especially through moments of uncertainty (see Table 9.1).[5] We developed an initial set of principles based on MPact's historical experience (see About the Evaluation). We assessed their utility through the evaluation data we collected throughout the project and in end-of-project reflection and learning exercises conducted with our partners in Rwanda in December 2019. Among the principles of practice that mattered the most in making progress on the ground, collaboration proved itself at the core (Chapter 6). When partners sought out allies with whom they shared common cause and made partners who complemented their strengths, their work blossomed. The very best among these collaborations, and those that endured beyond Project ACT, were characterized by reciprocal learning and by aligned action. Strong allied partnerships proved so vital to forward momentum, that where they were not central components of the local approach, the work proceeded in fits and starts, barely rising off the ground.

The principle of explicit accountability to human rights also undergirded the successes we observed. Human rights were central to the framings in the materials partners developed, the training sessions that they designed and conducted, the legal and policy analyses they performed, and to each of the other tactics they deployed. Adherence to a human rights framework was readily apparent in how the partners sought to hold those who held power by virtue of their professional roles to account for protecting sexual and gender minority constituents' right to health. Explicitly attempting to leverage the entry points to the policies and practices that create structural barriers, and, in some cases, elevating the ability of young gay men and

Table 9.1 Project ACT Principles

Collaborate	Seek out allies with whom you share a common cause and partners who complement your strengths. Seek regular opportunities to learn from their successes, failures, and challenges. Ensure your actions are aligned with the actions of your allies.
Observe human rights frameworks	Question and challenge the fundamental inequalities promoted by mainstream and government institutions. Hold duty-bearers and others who hold power by virtue of their professional role to account for protecting the right to health for all sexual and gender minority people. Facilitate the participation of all sexual and gender minority people in society based on their fundamental human rights. Leverage the entry points to the laws, policies, and practices that create structural barriers to health care access for sexual and gender minority people.
Empower	Nurture others' leadership potential by assisting them to gain the skills and the experiences required to advocate. Facilitate their linkages to peers and allied communities and institutions. Continually create opportunities for them to engage in strategic initiatives. Reinforce and nurture their strengths.
Remain agile	Adapt to changes in the field, shifting tactics as necessary to achieve strategic objectives and minimize harm to your constituency. Capitalize on unexpected opportunities to advance your agenda.
Tailor to the context	Regularly conduct crosscutting political and socio-structural analysis. Choose tactics appropriate to your agenda and analysis of local conditions. Frame languages and messages to suit the local context.
Use evidence	Incorporate the best available evidence from credible sources into campaigns. To the best of your ability, fill gaps in the evidence that is available.
Protect the safety of staff and constituents	Assess risks to the safety and security of all involved. Make every effort to mitigate those risks. Inform campaign workers and constituents of likely risks and risk mitigation procedures. Identify the probability of backlash and other negative responses to campaigns that might increase constituents' vulnerability in society or set back current efforts. Weigh the probable benefits and costs of planned actions in light of the probability of potential damage to constituents and the larger mission.
Strive for inclusion	Prioritize the needs and concerns of the most marginalized and excluded rather than of the most privileged community members on whose behalf you are working. Incorporate the perspective of those who are most impacted by oppression and whose rights are most under threat into your advocacy efforts and the process for setting and revising your agenda.
Routinely reflect	Engage in routine reflection on and reassessment of strategies and tactics. Engage in critical reflection and team dialogue throughout all phases of project planning, implementation, and closure. Create opportunities for dissent and deliberative dialogue with constituents.
Respect others	Strive to honor and respect the dignity and self-worth of others. Honor and respect local knowledge and expertise.

transgender women to participate in civil society processes, also demonstrates the role of the principle of human rights in guiding partners toward successful outcomes.

Attention to empowerment—a closely related principle—also proved essential (Chapter 5). The empowerment principle showed itself clearly in the value added of the systematic cultivation of the leadership of young gay and bisexual men and transgender women, attention paid to nurturing nascent institutions led by these community members, and provision of meaningful advocacy opportunities to them. Dymond in Jamaica, Thea in Cameroon, and Blessing and Siphosenkosi in Zimbabwe are only four among more than 20 others from Project ACT whom we might have highlighted individually. Empowering actions provided healing and connection (Chapter 5) and, as Christens indicates (2021), disrupted the consciousness of powerlessness created by living in a stigmatizing environment.

Partners' successes also depended on their agility. Partners' manner of responding to the challenges they encountered by shifting tactics and reacting quickly to changes in their environment (Chapter 7) points to their agility. MPact played an important role in facilitating adherence to a principle of agility by exercising tremendous flexibility over workplans, in response to events on the ground, and by welcoming the constant reevaluation of how best to remove barriers to HIV health care, promote equity, and mitigate the structural inequities that disadvantage gay and bisexual men and transgender women in each country.

Additional principles, evidenced in speaking to journalists, health care workers, and others, is the use of sound evidence as a component of advocacy messaging. Data prompted these people to act. The incorporation of mystery patient data collection to generate data where it was lacking captured the attention of advocacy targets and those who the partners desired to cultivate as champions. Coupling evidence with the sensitization training programs centered in contemporary science on human sexuality and reflective of social psychological knowledge on perspective taking proved a potent combination, as noted earlier. The use of tactics that took account of cultural norms, such as how one interacts appropriately with elders (Chapter 5) and how best to address sensitive topics, also helped activists gain entry and, ultimately, traction.

Project ACT provides lessons, too, about principles that should have provided stronger guides to the activists. When Project ACT faltered, essential principles of sound advocacy practice were not in the fore. Perhaps the most surprising principle given short shrift was safety, which received too limited attention and critical analysis as part of workplan development. Assessing the risks to the safety and security of everyone involved and mitigating those risks was a limited aspect of the project's planning process (Chapter 4). Insufficient time was devoted to critically analyzing workplans for foreseeable backlash, negative responses, and the increased vulnerability that using certain tactics was likely to cause. The "what if" component of planning, when absent, leaves activists vulnerable. It is not entirely clear whether the Project ACT partners simply accept the risks of the work that they do as a matter of course, or simply approach safety reactively. Probably both. Safety in advocacy, as Project ACT helps show, is not limited to risks such as violent backlash and government interference. Risks related to stress, mental health, and reputation are also present. Anticipating these risks as part of the cost of advocacy and developing plans to address them is wise. Systems of support, healing, and care are essential components of safety, just as they are a prerequisite for empowerment. That said, in some contexts, the options for contingencies are very limited and heavily constrained by the structural nature of stigma, by classism, and by neocolonialism. These structural barriers to safety must also be torn down.

In addition to limited attention given to the principle of safety, at least until it became unavoidable and demanded action in the field, a lack of community inclusion hurt the work in some countries.[6] Recovering from unanticipated challenges in Cameroon, for example, came about through a rapid pivot to a community-centered and inclusive model of planning and operation. Bringing people together turned things around. Local critics of the work in other countries pointed to noninclusive approaches as limiting. It cannot be taken for granted that working in a community-led organization is equivalent to having in place systematic and routine processes for hearing from and taking serious account of the perspectives of those who are most impacted by oppression and whose rights are most under threat. Those who work in community-led organizations may be among more privileged community members rather than among the most marginalized and excluded (Chapter 2). The tensions we uncovered among transgender people in gay-led organizations are a case in point.[7] Operating from the principle of inclusion encourages activists to continuously reflect on the complicated diversity of their community and their own position and privileges within it. It also helps them to understand how their biases are reflected in the issues they put forward as advocacy priorities (which is perhaps what makes this principle so difficult to enact). Inclusion may also help activists to devise advocacy plans that take account of the risks and threats their work poses to members of the community who are least like themselves. Project ACT showed many of the partners that acting on this principle had the potential to enhance the relevance and quality of their work. Identifying these advocacy principles—safety and inclusion—extends the work of Christens (2021) in establishing a compelling list of design principles for pursuing social change and enhancing community power.

The Value and Principles of Transnational Alliances

A second question we set out to explore concerned what, if anything, a transnational partner like MPact meaningfully contributes to local advocacy results. Did this work really require a unified vision and centralized coordination, support, and resources? Answering this question always felt to Robin as the most politically troublesome, if for no other reason than this was a question of central interest to the LGBT Fund but not to MPact; MPact, as George conveys in Chapter 3, was confident of its approach, while also eager to learn through evaluation how it might do its work more effectively.

We both knew all along that MPact's model struck people at the LGBT Fund as probably not worth its cost. Robin also feared their skepticism could be well placed. Why pass money through a group like MPact? Given known limitations of implementing partners from Global North countries (Chapter 2), why engage one to oversee this sort of work?

Part of answering this question lies in an understanding of MPact's underlying mission in relationship to the dynamics of power and vulnerability in which community-led organizations are trapped. At its heart, MPact aims to empower the people associated with nascent sexual and gender minority community-led organizations throughout the world to secure control over their lives and affairs. Its activities are meant to catalyze others' ability to advocate for what they need and desire. MPact hopes to ensure that activists are coordinated in their actions, which can help prevent powerful actors from pitting organizations against one another and sowing divisions among them. They leverage their own relationships to break down barriers to others' access to power. This is the essence of what an organization like MPact tries to bring to efforts like Project ACT.

Did they? It is unsurprising, given that MPact's role is to enable other activists to gain power, that when Robin asked the partners direct questions about MPact's contributions to their work, they often paused. They rightly hesitated to give MPact credit for their efforts and achievements. Indeed, they couldn't. At first, they would express uncertainty, or they might talk about money. But in their informal interactions with Robin, they answered this question repeatedly and clearly without her ever posing it. The direct interventions that MPact made to secure an audience with an official or access resources were easy to point to in our casual conversations. These contributions to the local work were plainly evident in most countries, and the partners from Burundi, Cameroon, Ghana, Jamaica, República Dominicana, and Zimbabwe made mention more than once that their local work benefited from these types of intervention. MPact's contributions also included the creation of and linkages to leadership ladders. Dymond's participation in training to start a pre-exposure prophylaxis (PrEP) demand campaign among transgender women and her competing successfully for a start-up grant to support her campaign were opportunities that MPact created. Partners found leadership bridges like these transformational and synergistic with the work they did via Project ACT. For Dymond, the PrEP demand workshop was a highlight moment in her growth as an activist. It bolstered her confidence. It also opened a new advocacy agenda at TransWave and at J-FLAG.[8] MPact's continual scanning of the international environment to ensure that its partners were aware of opportunities and had access to them was a valued contribution to the local work. Partners appreciated MPact's ongoing effort to make sure that they gained access to professional development, significant meetings, and influential networks.

MPact's contributions to local work also came through its direct engagement in skill development activities in the Cambodia and Rwanda workshops, and through site visits to partner countries. For those who attended it, the Cambodia workshop was a seminal learning event, in addition to its contribution to forging enduring connections among the partners. Although the workshop was flawed in certain respects (Chapter 4), its value to the partners far outweighed its limitations. In the workshop, participants learned how to do things such as map power and identify leverage points in the systems they aspired to influence. This was one of several aspects of advocacy planning that proved novel for many of the partners. The workshops cultivated skills and introduced tools that the partners were excited to use in their work.

When the MPact staff site-visited their partners, they reached beyond the organizational leaders who came to Cambodia and Rwanda, ensuring that skills and advice were directly transmitted to the local staff and collaborators. For instance, this was a critical component of developing advocacy champions among health care workers in Zimbabwe. On-the-ground visits permitted MPact to join partners in meetings with local officials. MPact staff's presence helped "grease the wheels" and call needed attention to the partners' work. In these latter engagements, partners also had the opportunity to directly observe the MPact staff members' advocacy skills. Partners perceived that their advocacy skills were cultivated in useful ways through on-site engagement. Reflecting on these occasions, partners said that their eyes were opened to new possibilities; their imagination and ambition enhanced. The partners' keenest wish, repeated interview after interview, was for more time spent with the MPact staff on developmental site visits. This, too, was among the MPact staff's sense of where they fell short of their own aspirations. They had too few on-the-ground engagements. Visits were too often timed to fit the MPact staff members' schedules, rather than timed when they might be most useful to a partner. Inconsistencies in providing technical assistance, and in the depth and breadth of what was offered across the countries, also topped the MPact staff's list of regrets. Even so, MPact's contributions to its partners' work are significant. It is easy to trace the actions MPact staff members took to leverage relationships and opportunities and to build skills to specific achievements at the country level.

Emphasizing day-to-day technical assistance actions, leadership development, mentorship, leveraging opportunities and access, and project coordination overshadows what Robin came to recognize as another of MPact's meaningful contributions to the local work: promoting the principle of a reflective advocacy practice. The more Robin became part of the team, the more often she had occasion to witness their transparency and routine of critical reflection. Gatherings at their home base in Oakland centered on self-reflection and team reflection. Their clarity around a collective vision supported them well in their reflective practices. What the staff believed was lacking in their individual and collective efforts and what they wanted to do differently was as much in the fore of discussion as what they thought they were getting right. They knew themselves well, both as individuals and as a team. Their candor and vulnerability were striking. They knew what they should do better. They adjusted as they went, taking concrete actions born out of their habits of reflection and an openness to trying alternatives. They used the evaluation results consistently. They developed a formal plan for how to work differently in the future based on what they learned through Project ACT's evaluation.

That same principle of reflection guided routine conversations between country leads and the in-country team members with whom they worked. These conversations occurred at least once a month, but often, more frequently. These regular meetings allowed the partners to brainstorm, problem-solve, obtain advice, and change directions, without restriction or fear of being told what they must do. Partners characterized these conversations as imbued with a respect for their expertise and local knowledge. The conversations provided partners with space and time to think, the value of which they quickly came to appreciate. It was in this way that MPact honored local values and infused a decolonizing stance into their approach.

MPact brought their culture of reflection with them to the project wrap-up meeting in Rwanda, a 3-day taking-stock workshop they held for all partners. Robin helped in its design and facilitation. The workshop drew on evaluative techniques that included storytelling, drawing, and appreciative inquiry methods (see About the Evaluation). The MPact team modeled reflective practices throughout the workshop, participating in the exercises themselves. As always, Robin took field notes. Partners frequently commented that they rarely take the time to take stock and reflect, as the MPact team was encouraging them to do. They stated emphatically that they valued the spaces MPact created throughout the project for this type of reflection and sharing. They wished there were more forums for cross-national learning to occur throughout the project and for those in the project who chose to implement similar tactics or target the same systems of power to share experiences. When Robin read the sheets hanging on the walls that summarized the lessons they were taking away from the project, she read observations such as "reflection provides an invaluable opportunity to enhance understanding of how meaningful accomplishments are produced," and "integrating evaluation, learning, and reflection enhances advocacy and helps move it forward." In one of the discussions, consensus quickly emerged that by embedding evaluation activities into the work all along, and by creating special spaces reserved to step back and think, MPact had granted its partners an opportunity to learn things that surprised them.

Fitting Evaluation to Context and Purpose

We intended our evaluation of Project ACT to meaningfully support (not in a tokenistic sense), respect (not in a performative sense), and generously give back to communities with which we feel a deep connection and whose goals we believe in. Communities we love. We were open about our assumptions, as we are open about them in this book, including our moral position on the right to health and well-being of sexual and gender minority communities, and our belief in the importance of their gaining power to shape, contribute to, and reside happily within the communities in which they live. For us, part of what this means is that the stakes in getting the advocacy right are exceedingly high, high enough that neither of us believes that simply because an effort is community-led, it is well done or worthwhile. Rather, we believe that what communities do deserves investment and study.

At the same time, we were open about the evaluation dilemmas we were struggling with (see Chapter 4) and dilemmas regarding the dynamics of Global North–Global South partnerships (Chapter 2), dilemmas that we still puzzle over and which writing this book has brought to the fore. Among the things that we learned through Project ACT was that we cannot escape the reality of our liberal values, our advantaged social positions, or our North American upbringings. These shape how we think and see the world. Instead, rather than accomplish the impossible task of shedding entirely who we are, what we can create is a setting in which we are free to discuss our challenges openly with our partners and invite them to challenge our actions, our values, and our interpretations and understandings of events. We can create a space for others to express their values, including those we find troublesome. When we succeed, they, too, find space to share their perspectives. Or at least that is what we, as outsiders who desire to be good partners to those who differ from us in innumerable ways, hope.

In our approach to the evaluation of Project ACT, we married the contemporary thinking on human rights and advocacy evaluation (e.g., Arensman, 2020; Arensman & van Wesel, 2018; Schlangen & Coe, 2021) with transformative practices rooted in the African context (e.g., Chilisa & Malunga, 2012; Chilisa & Mertens, 2021; Mertens, 2009). The principles emerging in the arena of LGBT evaluation (e.g., Phillips et al., 2022) were also tested in this process. Although every evaluator might merge these perspectives and principles differently, our integration, including its search for useful principles of advocacy practice, its harvesting of outcomes, and its ongoing feeding back of information, created a learning structure that ensured the engagement of the Project ACT team in its design and implementation. It was fit for its purpose.

Evaluation practitioners have only recently begun to articulate approaches to evaluation that are appropriate to and can contribute to human rights advocacy (Chapter 4). These approaches are generally subsumed under the growing specialization of advocacy evaluation, which has pushed evaluators toward the development of evaluations that are suitable to complex situations. They draw on a general movement toward complexity-informed evaluation practices (see, for example, Schwandt & Gates, 2021). Human rights evaluation—a distinct subtype of these approaches—is contribution focused. It orients itself toward using evaluations to understand human rights advocacy's contributions to change and illuminating how changes happen. It takes account of what reflects meaningful progress in context and from a community perspective. A central goal of the approach is to assist activists to learn; to inform their choice of immediate and future advocacy strategies. Its uniqueness comes, in part, from its explicit moral grounding, its sensitivity to safety and security considerations, and its expectation that advocacy campaigns invite resistance because they challenge entrenched inequities in structural power. These insights inform methodological choices and temper understandings of achievement. Human rights evaluation positions the evaluator as a steward of the human rights advocacy efforts they study. Although serving as steward may not fully address every dilemma that we identify in Chapter 4, it provides the evaluator with a north-star guiding principle when encountering inevitable practice dilemmas.

Whereas human rights advocacy evaluation is a new development in practice, LGBTQ + evaluation as a formalized approach to practice is newer still. Robin's life work as an evaluator (Miller, 2018) and our experiences evaluating Project ACT (Miller, 2021; Miller & Tohme, 2022) inform the sole framework in this emerging practice arena (Felt et al., 2024; Phillips et al., 2022, 2023). Emerging out of the culturally responsive and equitable evaluation movements (e.g., Dean-Coffey et al., 2014; Donaldson & Picciotto, 2016; Hood et al., 2015; Hopson & Cram, 2018; Kirkhart, 2010; SenGupta et al., 2004) and the Transformative Paradigm (Mertens, 2009), LGBTQ + evaluation offers a principles-driven framework to guide practice. These principles call for evaluations that are informed by historical and contemporary dynamics of sexual and gender minority oppression, give priority to allyship with sexual and gender minority communities, encourage decolonial practice, and privilege community ownership and leadership over evaluation processes, among other principles.

Through enacting a style of evaluation rooted in human rights frameworks and by using advocacy-appropriate methods, not only did we document project achievements and desirable advocacy outcomes at the country level, but we also uncovered principles and bore witness to advocacy enacted. We showed how advocacy exerted pressure on duty bearers—the holders of power who are responsible for realizing rights (e.g., repealing punitive laws, rewriting harmful policies, changing discriminatory practices that maintain inequities and thwart connectedness to self and community). Power and principles are threads that link the stories we share on the pages of this book. Every chapter illustrates systems of power—the power of funders, the power of health care professionals, the power of government officials and policymakers, the power of evaluators (why George was afraid of Robin looking so deeply and intimately at the workings of MPact),[9] and most importantly, the power of community to mobilize and apply pressure for change.

Project ACT Revisited

Projects like Project ACT are not always politically palatable to funders. Just as occurs within the well-bounded conventional projects in which funders typically invest, donors to advocacy have power to dictate the terms and degree of an advocacy effort. By the terms that they set, they may curb the degree of responsiveness to community concerns. They may restrict the latitude to pursue what local people believe is important. They may starve communities of sufficient money to do the work. Although Project ACT, through MPact's leadership, pushed back against this tendency in its design and execution, the project was stunted by an insultingly short time frame and small budget. That the partners accomplished what they did in such an underfunded circumstance, and so quickly, is its own miracle. The modesty of Project ACT's budget limited not just its scope of accomplishment, but its evaluation, too.[10] Indeed, the evaluation work we accomplished depended substantially on the in-kind contributions of Michigan State University. It also depended on Robin's ability and willingness to donate most of her time as an unpaid laborer to this effort and to use faculty research funds to supplement the available budget. [11] She recruited ample volunteer labor from students. Without all these in-kind contributions, the evaluation simply could not have been done. In one of Robin's meetings in Cameroon, an official asserted that evaluation was, in her view, not worth its outrageous price tag. We can only hope this modest evaluation, fueled principally by donated resources and effort, proves her assertion wrong. For George, only after we partnered in writing this book, did he realize that there was never any real interest in Project ACT on the part of its funders, let alone the evaluation efforts upon which this book is based. The LGBT Fund press conference (Chapter 3) makes sense to George now in an entirely new way: What his funder only really cared about was settling a debt they felt they owed to MPact. A decolonized approach to funding efforts like Project ACT suggests that donors must learn not to think of themselves as more important than those whom they fund. George's staff were pushed to take on more work than they could handle to pull off Project ACT, to go above and beyond what the funder required to ensure their partners' success.

We set out on a journey to evaluate an innovative and coordinated set of advocacy initiatives led by sexual and gender minority people living in Africa and the Caribbean to reduce the stigma, discrimination, and violence that impedes their access to HIV health care. We desired to build on a thin knowledge base about what advocacy practice in this arena requires and to explore evaluation practices that support it. We gathered evidence that might illuminate how and why local sexual and gender minority-led organizations working in partnership with principled transnational peers are critical to sexual and gender minority people, to their health access, to their connectedness, to their human rights, to their survival. And to ours. The account we have offered of Project ACT in this book reveals the beautifully messy and deliberate process inherent to human rights advocacy, and to engaged scholarship itself. Project ACT highlights the vital role of sexual and gender minority community-led organizations in changing their local systems of health care, of transnational partnerships in supporting these local efforts at structural change, and the role evaluation can play in these contexts.

Epilogue

Robin

I never observed Cameroon's majesty from the sky. My flights from Paris always landed shortly after dusk, descending through the dense layers of thunderclouds that formed over the jungle during the afternoon heat. The occasional flicker of lights is fleeting as the plane passes downward over the mountains that ring the basin in which Cameroon's capital city sits. Landing in Yaoundé at night always stimulates my sense of hypervigilance. I am one of few pale-skinned Westerners disembarking the plane. Stone-faced officials control the multiple health and passport screenings I pass through. I wait in a throng of sweat-drenched passengers, who squeeze around a creaking carousel as it churns with overstuffed suitcases, some taped at their midsections, others spewing their contents onto the belt. Uniformed men hugging machine guns patrol the terminal and its roadway checkpoints. I am slow to gain my bearings in these unfamiliar surroundings, especially at night.

Bastien steers us toward Yaoundé through the inky darkness of deserted lowland forests, along twisting clay roads that abruptly disintegrate into cavernous ruts. Once beyond the immediate surrounds of the airport, in its heavily guarded isolation, and speeding down the 23 miles of disorienting bends and curves toward the heart of the city, Yaoundé pulsates with the business of the nighttime streets, revealed at first only in shadows cast by strings of lights hanging above roadside stalls and in open-air grilles. Isolated spots of vibrant activity gradually become conjoined, until people seem to move as one along the roadside. The dusty, rutted arteries branching out from the city's heart teem with people. They idle together in partial shadow under dimly lit canopies, sharing platters of grilled plantains. They tote packages and baskets atop their heads and dozing children on their backs. The liveliness passing by my window in this incredible place does little to ease my somber feelings. My visits to Yaoundé are always tinged by the sobering realization that the work performed by the people I am there to see is as dangerous as it is significant. That any one of the people I observe going about their nightly business from the windows of the battered Toyota van I ride in might seek to harm my colleagues without pause or concern.[1] That the activists of Project ACT might be endangered in the very communities they love and consider their home unsettles me in ways that I doubt I will ever move past.

Evaluating Project ACT deepened my understanding of what the activists in the project confront each day, the steepness of the perilous hills they are climbing together, and the tremendous risks they bear to recreate their societies as just and loving places for sexual and gender minority people. As an evaluator, it is a delicate balance to strike to act as a co-steward of their work and serve in the role of their critical friend, while remaining sensitive to the fact that I am an outsider in every sense. I am acutely aware of how very much of an outsider I am on every trip, no matter how graciously and warmly welcomed I feel. I can never know what it is like to do my colleagues' work, day in and day out; to live with its hazards, trials, joys, and triumphs. I only know what people chose to show and tell me. They will only share so much. And I can only understand what they share through the lenses of someone who lives in a world of different challenges, possibilities, and privileges. Observing the nighttime streets of Yaoundé through the windows of Bastien's speeding van always recalls this to me.

I flew out of Yaoundé for the final time just before midnight on Saturday, March 7, 2020, with a quick turnaround to my next Project ACT site. I was bound for Kingston, Jamaica, to meet with Dymond, Akoni, and Jaden. Immediately afterward, I was to head to Bulawayo, Zimbabwe, for my final visit with Mandla, Mbuso, and the local team. I was unable to visit all the places I needed to; my graduate student, Jaleah, was due to depart for Accra in a week to learn more about how mystery patients were deployed and received in Ghana. The MPact Project ACT team and I were in a furious rush to complete our work by the grant deadline of March 31. Our final reports were due June 1. For our partners, for all intents and purposes, Project ACT was over, prematurely so. Everyone understood the stakes tied to the evaluation of the project. Most had told me time after time how important it was to continue the advocacy started under the project. We knew what strategies needed refinement, scaling, and more comprehensive evaluation. The people I met in Cameroon were most insistent on this point. Project ACT stimulated something momentous in Yaoundé that must be nurtured, they told me. Although the Cameroonians expressed this belief most forcefully, it is fair to say that from Dymond to Mandla to Claude to Halima, everyone believed in the value of their partnership with MPact and in the continuation of Project ACT. They said plainly that the work we had started must be sustained. Their allies and constituents agreed. We all knew what ought to happen next.

The day before I left Cameroon, I made one last visit to Central Hospital, the second of the week, to observe the presentation of certificates of excellence to the day clinic staff. As our truck maneuvered through the busy campus, we found it transformed. Every one of the hospital's personnel wore a mask. None had before. When we entered the day hospital, we learned that Cameroon's first COVID-19 patient, a French traveler, was somewhere in the facility. A physician whom I had interviewed earlier in the week urged me to wear a mask when I transferred planes in Paris. When I returned to my hotel in the late afternoon, the personnel there were wearing masks. None had done so when I left in the morning. Guests were required to use hand sanitizer before and after the metal detector security screening to enter the building. Although I sensed the high anxiety of the physicians and hotel staff, I could not have anticipated that the day before I was to leave for Jamaica, my university would suspend international travel indefinitely and, quickly thereafter, domestic travel, even within the state. Project ACT's evaluation came to an abrupt stop, as did nearly everything else in the world.

It quickly became clear that Project ACT's evaluation must finish out in an entirely virtual fashion, to the extent that was possible. It was not. Our partners in Zimbabwe do not have the Internet infrastructure or predictable access to electricity to support virtual engagement. They were locked down, too, limiting their communications locally, so much of which ordinarily occur face to face, person to person. What proved possible was a meager substitute for the on-the-ground data collection: WhatsApp calls. The MPact team and I waded into a new world of interactive virtual meetings on Zoom, culling our lessons learned through these less-than-optimal virtual means of communication, and learning how to use these tools as we stumbled along. Suffice it to say, virtual communications miserably fail to replicate the culture of closeness, proximity, and community that characterizes how each of the Project ACT organizations normally functions.

Although we succeeded in making our way through these final activities and managed a bare minimum of long-distance data collection with partners in Zimbabwe, Jamaica, and Ghana, MPact's plan to sustain the work suffered most under COVID-19. Its negotiation with the LGBT Fund over a sustainability concept was paused, given an unclear future driven by the emergence of a new global pandemic, and the desire of the Fund to shuffle its portfolio in response. Time under lockdown passed. And as it passed, many of the partners to Project ACT moved through transformations driven by shifts in funding patterns reflecting inattention to HIV, by lockdowns that necessitated changing how HIV activists and outreach teams worked to ensure ongoing access to HIV testing and care services under the worst possible circumstances, and by the many ordinary organizational and personal events that change organizations. The country contexts shifted, too, with upticks in repression occurring in Cameroon and Ghana, as in other parts of Africa. Although traces of the work begun under Project ACT remain evident in several organizations, we are not in a position to assess the project's long-term legacy. MPact changed immensely during these years, too. Its staffing and direction changed. It is pursuing new things. In the end, as too often occurs, Project ACT part II never happened.

I had my final conversation with Emil late on the Friday afternoon of March 6, 2020, the day before I left Cameroon for the last time. He reflected on the lessons he had taken away from Project ACT. He had always believed that health care providers had sworn an oath of beneficence and would adhere to it. In Project ACT, he learned just how severely bias undermines that oath. Health care providers, he observed, are prisoners of their culture. "Nothing should be taken for granted," he concluded. "We need to update them constantly." Earlier that same week, I met with a Cameroonian official who oversees a health district serving about 1 million people via 245 facilities, a district with the highest estimated HIV prevalence among gay and bisexual men in the country: 40%–45%. His district suffers immense gaps in HIV testing and care, exacerbated by constant collapses in supply chains. When I asked him what lessons he had learned from Project ACT, he said, "It is possible even in the face of expected resistance. Work with people in the field from the bottom up," he advised. "Just do it as a call to conscience. This project was a beginning."

George

In the weeks before its end, the team and I elaborated a new plan to continue Project ACT. Our plan would scale up our work in Cameroon and Zimbabwe, bring Project ACT to new countries in Africa, and test its concept in Asia. But, as the COVID-19 pandemic raged on, as hard as we tried, we were unsuccessful. HIV was no longer top of mind for donors. Funders shifted their attention. The opportunity to pursue our vision faded. COVID-19 was just one of several pressures international funders felt to redirect their resources. Europe and North America were grappling with heated border control debates while addressing the needs of displaced peoples. Support for international, community-led advocacy focused on the needs of sexual and gender minority people seemed to slip further and further down the priority list. This spelled trouble for organizations like MPact. I knew that MPact would need ties to unrestricted donor gifts. That kind of funding could only be gotten through relationships with pharmaceutical companies and monied people. I did not possess the social capital to permit me entrée into those circles. My relationships just did not extend in those directions. When it came to money and mainstream celebrity, I was not an A-Gay. MPact needed something different.

I left MPact in the fall of 2020. My body was tired. My partner was tired. My heart hurt. I needed to spend more time taking care of myself, my relationship, my parents, my home. Many of the staff at MPact also left to pursue their passions in other organizations. Stephen. Mohan. Nadia. Greg. Omar. Johnny. And other champions who diligently, passionately worked in the background to ensure Project ACT's success. All staff members from my time with the organization have since moved on. Don Baxter stayed a member of the MPact board of directors another 9 months after my departure. Long enough to see a new executive director named and to pass the board chair role over to his successor. MPact's new executive director called me regularly during his early days at MPact. I was happy to support in any way I could. Still am. The calls are much less frequent now. That is OK. A good sign, I suppose. I'm uncertain whether MPact held its relationships with the Project ACT partners. I like to imagine that MPact retains respectful, meaningful, and well-funded advocacy partnerships in Africa and the Caribbean, especially in countries where HIV prevalence remains high and access to HIV services remains obstructed by punitive laws and policies. But the funding ecosystem is parched. And MPact is a different place, nearly unrecognizable to me now. I do not look back.

In 2021, the latest year for which we have complete data, 1.5 million people globally were newly infected with HIV (UNAIDS, 2022a). The COVID-19 pandemic is, no doubt, partly to blame. That same year, in sub-Saharan Africa, "key populations" accounted for 51% of new HIV infections and 70% of all new infections globally. Dramatic increases. We are heading in the wrong direction. Modelers have estimated that progress made in our global response to HIV has been set back 10 years due to COVID-19. The loss of progress is staggering. All while violence directed at sexual and gender minority people remains pervasive and anti-homosexuality laws stand in Burundi, Cameroon, Ghana, Jamaica, and Zimbabwe. The year 2021 is also distinguished as the deadliest on record for trans, gender queer, and nonbinary people, with 375 documented murders of transgender people worldwide. Advocacy and other community tactics to tear down barriers to HIV services for sexual and gender minority people were and continue to be urgently needed. We need transnational advocacy organizations led by gay and bisexual men and transgender people. We need MPact, perhaps more now than ever before. I leave it to readers to judge whether Project ACT shows why these organizations and transnational coordination by peer activists remain vital and deserving of support.

Appendix

About the Evaluation

When George and I initially established the plan for my guest year with MPact, we agreed I would examine how MPact and its global partners conducted evaluations and assess the quality of those evaluations by conducting a metaevaluation.[1] We also agreed I would help George develop a simple self-evaluation framework for MPact and its partners' use. Our plan was discarded when George hit on the idea of my evaluating Project ACT (Chapter 4). The evaluation I conducted and the observations I made of the Project ACT team form the evidentiary base for this book.

The development of the evaluation took months of effort. The most intense period of its development occurred between August and December 2018. Nadia, an MPact staff member and the project lead, served as my liaison. She had no experience of commissioning and managing an evaluation. After we all came home from the 2018 IAS Conference in Amsterdam (Chapter 4), I created a generic task list for her on planning and managing an evaluation. One column outlined evaluator responsibilities and another staff responsibilities, along with a timeline. I sent the task list to her by email, along with a note indicating that we were woefully behind. At that point, advocacy was underway in some countries. We had missed the window to obtain baseline assessments. We had not determined evaluation questions, approaches, or methods. To catch up, I proposed that I come out for a planning week in Oakland. Nadia responded immediately, "Come in 2 weeks, dear."

My advance work for that week included conducting 15 semistructured interviews with the MPact team and others associated with MPact, a few of the leaders of the Project ACT partner organizations, and a handful of representatives from MPact donor organizations. This advance work was especially important because my part of the agenda in Cambodia was truncated to address higher priority topics (Chapter 4). Inspired by appreciative inquiry techniques (Coghlan et al., 2003),[2] I had constructed an exercise that culminated in our partners identifying three wishes to make the monitoring and evaluation of Project ACT useful to move advocacy forward, remove obstacles, and enable achievements. We had no time for it. Instead, these semistructured interviews would inform our decision making.

I began each interview by asking people to imagine two alternative scenarios. In the first, Project ACT had achieved successes beyond anyone's wildest imagination. I told them to imagine that we were gathering for a fabulous party in London at the Elton John AIDS Foundation headquarters to celebrate our achievements. I then asked them to tell me what had happened to bring us together. In the second scenario, I asked them to imagine their nightmare alternative: We had returned to

Cambodia to conduct a postmortem on the disastrous consequences of Project ACT. Again, I asked them to describe what had occurred that led to our funeral gathering. After obtaining these two alternative visions, I asked them to consider the more likely scenarios that lay between their terrifying and triumphant fantasies. I asked them to identify the questions that they thought must be answered by an evaluation, and to tell me why each question was important. I also asked if resources permitted that only one question could be addressed, which was most important to them. We discussed who might be positively and negatively impacted by the evaluation. I sought their advice on how to make the evaluation successful. I concluded by asking them to identify three hopes for the project's ultimate success.

Person by person, I acquired a rich list of the potential negative consequences of the work, aspirations for it, and important constituencies whose experience and perspective I must consider. I learned what kinds of information the people who would use the evaluation required and what they were especially curious about. I could determine where the donors, the partners, and the MPact staff and leadership converged and diverged in their reasons for wanting an evaluation, and in their hopes and fears. I was struck by points of convergence. The MPact staff and project partners believed that a principal reason to conduct an evaluation was that advocacy is "so ridiculously hard to pin down," yet they all believed that when activist communities work together, "magic" can happen. They all perceived their work to be poorly understood. They often found it difficult to make the case for what they do because they lack conventional empirical proof of its value. Demonstrating the role activist communities play in the HIV response and painting a vivid portrait of their work were among their primary motivations for conducting an evaluation. An evaluation might help others understand what communities contribute and buttress arguments for increased support of community efforts. A member of the MPact staff expressed this shared perspective:

> Why is it important to have community involvement for accessing health care for LGBT people? There is a real disinvestment going on and no money for communities. I want to show why a sustainable community system is part of the HIV response. It feels like we are starting from scratch on this conversation about communities. I want concrete examples. I want life stories. I want to show how advocacy works.

One of the donors offered a similar view. They noted that, as a funder, their organization rarely has access to concrete details on what those that they fund do, and how the work that they support is situated within and appropriate to the local, national, or regional context:

> What does MPact and the partners really do on a day-to-day basis? We understand the big picture of how a program like this might be part of addressing big issues such as LGBT decriminalization, but as part of that, moving from the abstract

notion to a more concrete idea of X partner did this and Y partner did this and because of what they did, we have seen at least this small thing change. Or maybe it's impossible in a 2-year time frame to see concrete changes from their actions, but at least, this is what they do so that we could hope in the longer term that would mean X.

MPact's unusual model of operating in a dual role as funder and partner also piqued peoples' interests. MPact builds advocacy capacity, contributes to country-level advocacy, and disburses and oversees project funds for efforts like Project ACT. Documenting how this unique global partnership model might result in stronger LGBT human rights advocacy organizations struck several people as an especially intriguing area of investigation. Some of the donors wondered if the model's added value came via its contribution to cross learning. The African and Caribbean partners expressed curiosity about how MPact built capacity, and how it enabled peer-to-peer support and learning across countries and continents.

The scenarios that the MPact staff and partners offered to convey their highest aspirations also reflected shared visions of success. The first was that advocacy successfully advanced the goal of reducing stigma and discrimination. The second was that MPact had nurtured vibrant partnerships and cross-country conversations within and across world regions. The specifics of these dreams, however, were striking for their modesty: sexual and gender minority community-led organizations were able to converse with their governments, even in the most difficult country environments; sexual and gender minority community-led organizations could establish or improve relationships with the police; steps were taken to improve the odds health care staff are familiar with and observe appropriate protocols for providing care in a sensitive manner; the Project ACT partners exchanged best practices and learned from one another. No one harbored illusions of what could be achieved over Project ACT's brief timescale.

The worries that people expressed about the severe damage a project like this one might cause far exceeded what I typically hear when I ask people to imagine the worst. I always ask a question like this because I want people to be prepared if an evaluation's results are not favorable. A question like this also sensitizes me to the range of unintended consequences I might look for. Usually, people mention the possibility of being ineffectual or wasting money. Sometimes they say that the outcomes that truly matter will only reveal themselves so long after the evaluation has ended, that there is no possibility of my providing credible proof of their initiative's merit. For most of the MPact staff and their country partners, their greatest anxieties were about heightening vulnerability and contributing to substantial deterioration of forward progress. The following nightmare of an MPact staff member reflected this common concern:

Countries are shut down and there is a crackdown. CSOs [community service organizations] are forced to close up shop. They are no longer legal entities or able to secure resources. They took on too much risk. We pushed them too hard because we wanted results. We shrunk the advocacy space. We put them at risk. They can no longer legally exist. They know better than outsiders do what is reasonable and what is not, and we did not listen. We listened too much to stakeholders who don't know the context or the work.

The lack of control over the context, and the possibility that the environment was not yet suitable for Project ACT, factored heavily into fears of backlash and backward momentum. Capacity deficits, especially around safety and security and leveraging of allies, also concerned the staff and partners, given the steep challenges the project was likely to face:

We have a negative or damaged reputation, or our partners do. Our partners are unable to obtain the cooperation they need. Threats to the mental health and physical safety of partner and in-country LGBT people occur as a result of the work due to increased visibility. These kinds of outcomes might occur if people have not considered how to build their visibility carefully and wisely, if systems are not in place to address hostility, and if partners fail to draw on allies and those in-country collaborators who confer protection.

By contrast, donors' anxieties centered on the potential opportunity cost of supporting Project ACT rather than funding a direct service. Could the same money lead to more indirect and direct benefits if spent differently? Are intermediaries really needed? Why not fund partners directly? One donor, to my surprise, flatly disagreed that community-determined priorities merited pursuit or investigation at all. Despite contributing to Project ACT financially, their institution prefers to focus on indicators of "epidemic control." "[Our leadership], is not a fan of advocacy, however important it has been to historical advances in fighting the epidemic," they asserted. Advocacy was a "distraction" from the real work and pursuit of "true problems."

I used the interview results to create an interactive workshop for the MPact team to help us establish the focus of the evaluation and make preliminary decisions. I wrote out each evaluation question verbatim on an individual file card. I chose a distinct color card for each type of stakeholder: donor, collaborating partner, MPact staff, and so on. I placed a dot on the back of the card that contained the question of highest importance to each person. When the team assembled, I gave them each a set of cards, chosen at random. I instructed them to work as a team to sort the cards into thematically similar groups on my sticky wall. The staff stood before the turquoise sheet, sorting, debating, and reclassifying the cards until they were satisfied.

The staff had organized the questions into basic themes, which they labeled as follows: MPact's contributions to its partners and their successes; the qualities of partnerships; the nature of work on the ground; the consequences of advocacy; and the role of the context in shaping what occurs. Within each theme, I asked the group to identify similar questions and to place those together. I then asked that they remove any questions they believed were of low priority, given the constraints created by limited evaluation resources, or because they were impossible to answer. We put these in a "parking lot" on the right side of the sticky wall. When they were satisfied with their sorting, I revealed what the colors represented. I also explained that a card that had a dot on its back meant it was the highest priority question of the person who had posed it. Using boundary questions from Ulrich's critical systems heuristics (1994),[3] I guided the staff through a discussion of whether the questions in our parking lot, by their exclusion, might undermine the evaluation's ethicality, legitimacy, or credibility, or lead us to omit a point of view that we ought to reflect. The ensuing discussion focused primarily on a single question: What is the value added of MPact? The team took the question from the parking lot and put it back on the priority side of the sticky wall. After another round of review, the team was satisfied. Through this exercise and the vigorous discussions that it stimulated, we came to agree on an evaluation guided by a threefold purpose: to understand the nature of MPact's contribution to the advocacy results achieved by the Project ACT partners; to understand whether and how MPact contributed to growth in the advocacy capacity of the Project ACT partner organizations; and to identify core principles of effective practice for technical support provision and advocacy. We organized our questions in alignment with these purposes. We refined the language of the questions to ensure they were clear, unbiased, and reasonable. We also confirmed that it was feasible to answer them.

We next turned our attention to a stack of cards I had made that listed the constituencies who had a stake in the evaluation and the project. What role should each play? When should they be engaged and why? Through this discussion, we affirmed that the partners and MPact staff should collaborate on all aspects of the evaluation, and that these two groups were its primary users. We wanted each group to have a sense of ownership over the evaluation. We decided to activate our volunteer planning group (Chapter 4) to review our proposed purposes and questions. Were they sensible and useful to them? Johnny and Mohan took the lead, along with me, in liaising with the partner planning group. We finished out the day by determining roles for each of the other groups named on the cards.

I used the following morning to interview an ally who could help me anticipate issues in the field and warn me of potential landmines. But mostly, I read in preparation for facilitating our final planning discussion for that week. I knew the evaluation must draw on frameworks and approaches to evaluation that are suitable to advocacy and to the complex process of contributing to international development (e.g., Annie E. Casey Foundation, 2007; Arensman, 2020; Arensman et al., 2018, Arensman & van Wessel, 2018; Earl et al., 2001; Gardner & Brindis, 2017; Patton, 2018; Patton et al., 2015). I thought through the implications of core assumptions of advocacy evaluation, notably that attributing impacts to a single actor is inappropriate and that advocacy does not operate in isolation of other actors or of the political, social, economic, cultural, and legal environment in which it occurs. My interviews confirmed the latter point. Even though MPact chose countries because, in the grander scheme of things, few donors direct their attention there (Chapter 3), the project was not going to operate in a barren landscape. Moreover, initiatives like Project ACT intend to enhance the contributions of many actors in a bid to promote in-country ownership, empowerment, self-determination, and agency. The workplans MPact and their partners had finalized over the summer engaged a bevy of others: community-led organizations, clinics, hospitals, government entities, and media. The more that Project ACT succeeds, the more difficult it might be to isolate and trace MPact's influence on in-country outcomes. I had to call upon methods suitable to situations of dynamic complexity to understand the work and its anticipated and unanticipated consequences. I pondered the diverse tactics that each partner planned to employ and what I knew then about the unique country contexts in which each worked. I worried over what was feasible and realistic for them to achieve in a short time. I wanted to find a way for the partners' values and those of their constituents to hold a prominent place in the evaluation. I wanted an approach that respected the difficult and dangerous nature of human rights advocacy.

I became convinced that combining outcome harvesting (Wilson-Grau, 2018; Wilson-Grau & Britt, 2012) and principles-based evaluation (Patton, 2018) offered us appropriate strategies. These approaches are easily blended, adding to their appeal. By the point that we started seriously planning the evaluation, I had observed the MPact staff for 6 months. I had come to recognize that they were guided by an implicit set of principles on which they all appeared to agree. Certain principles recurred in their conversations and written products. Drawing these principles out made sense. They could serve as a rubric. We could examine whether and how these principles emerged in practice. We could identify others. We could understand the quality of the partnership through principles. We could understand effective advocacy through principles. That is precisely what a principles-based approach aims to do. It assumes that in the face of dynamic uncertainty, people navigate best when they have inspiring and useful principles to guide their decisions, rather than rigidly prescribed, inflexible recipes.

The uncertainties about what advocacy might produce in the eyeblink of 20 months was a commonly expressed concern. The MPact staff also worried that meaningful progress in one context may not look like very much had occurred in another. The logic and procedures of outcome harvesting suited these uncertainties and context-dependent understandings of meaningful change. Outcome harvesting is a rigorous method designed to capture outcomes in situations where there is uncertainty about what to expect and when changes might be observed. Outcome harvesting is also appropriate for determining if and how different actors may have contributed to observed changes. During a harvest, the evaluator works with evaluation participants to identify observed changes in how individuals and institutions behave. Changes may be positive or negative, beneficial or harmful, intended or unintended, expected or unexpected. Then, much like a detective, the evaluator gathers evidence to verify each change occurred and determine the extent to which an intervention (or actor) made a credible contribution to it. The harvest process includes a process for articulating why each outcome matters, which has the benefit of permitting local people to describe what they value and see as important. I worried that it might be difficult to convey to donors who are unfamiliar with the approach that it is incredibly rigorous.

Outcome harvesters carefully weigh the strength and breath of evidence, the plausibility and logic of interconnections, and thoroughly investigate alternative explanations to warrant their outcome claims. That very rigor compelled me to recommend we use the approach, given the skepticism about the value of advocacy expressed by some interviewees. When I explained the two approaches to the team, I was surprised at how excited the team was in response. The approaches made sense to them, too.

We now faced the arduous task of scaling down our ambitions to the evaluation's preliminary budget cap, which was far too small to support an evaluation of the scale we desired. George proposed that we select four partners to observe intensively over time. If we invested in studying just four partners' evolution and progress, he offered, we might gain more insight than if we studied every partner superficially. This struck us all as a worthwhile compromise. We set about deciding how to select which of the partners to observe. We started by considering the workplans and the variety of activities within them. But we kept returning to the matter of partnerships, their quality, and MPact's capacity-building mission. We ultimately settled on sorting the partners into quadrants along two dimensions: whether MPact had a short or long history working in the country, and whether the partner was a mature advocacy organization or early in the process of developing advocacy competence. We anchored each dimension and sorted the partners into one of the four resulting cells. Three of the cells contained two partners. For each of these cells, we discussed which of the two would be most feasible to study, considering factors such as country stability and the risk of increasing the activists' vulnerability to adverse outcomes through on-the-ground data collection. We prioritized observing the work in Cameroon, Côte d'Ivoire, Jamaica, and Zimbabwe. As it turned out, selecting these countries permitted us to cover the range from authoritarian to democratic governance, from economically fragile to stable, and from egregious to merely just inhospitably bad on LGBT human rights and hate-driven violence. We laid out a plan to convene our evaluation planning committee to weigh in on this part of our initial plan and, assuming this made sense to them, too, assist us with designing instruments and field and safety procedures. We proposed starting our work in Jamaica and asking our Jamaican partners if they were willing to help us by pilot testing our procedures and instruments. Doing so would give us time to translate and back-translate a final set of materials and secure visas for travel to Africa. Akoni agreed to my visiting Jamaica first.

I returned to Oakland 5 weeks later for a second week of planning. By that point, we had elaborated an evaluation workplan and timeline. Johnny and I had studied the pertinent data privacy laws in each country and their prohibitions on encryption software. He and I had also reviewed the current best practices on digital safety for human rights workers. I had touched base with the State Department's Division of Democracy, Human Rights and Labor for advice on our initial data security and country visit plans. I worked with my department's information technology expert to set up a system for safely transporting and storing digital information. I had applied for and received my institutional review board determination letter. Akoni and I had finalized our plan to test our site visit procedures and measures. I had reread each of MPact's annual reports, several white papers, and its current strategic plan. From these documents, I had extracted a candidate list of statements of principle that I could use as sensitizing concepts and in the development of interview guides and an online advocacy capacity survey to identify the partners' technical assistance needs. Johnny, Mohan, Greg, Omar, and I collapsed, added, revised, and rewrote that list until we felt ready to share our draft with George and Nadia. When Johnny exclaimed that he was going to hang our draft over his desk for inspiration, I took it as a sign we had succeeded in producing a relevant set of principles. We created a checklist for site visit preparation. We roughed out the contours of an ongoing communication plan, with routine touch points for the MPact team, the partners, and other stake- holders. With Pierre, Emil, Penya, Abou, and Claude's help, Johnny, Mohan, and I crafted a detailed strategy for site visits, including translator selection, safety precau- tions, data collection procedures, and other logistics. The eight of us outlined partner responsibilities for in-country data collection. We settled on a tentative schedule in which I would make three weeklong visits to Cameroon, Côte d'Ivoire, Jamaica, and Zimbabwe spaced out over a period of 15 months. We also committed to hold a wrap- up workshop to capture the experiences and lessons learned by all the partners.

I visited the partners we had selected for intensive study during my hemisphere's winter of 2018/19 and summer of 2019, beginning with that first trip to Jamaica on December 9, 2018. After revising our procedures, I traveled to Zimbabwe, Cameroon, and Côte d'Ivoire. I returned to the latter three countries in July and August 2019, postponing my second trip to Jamaica until September because Akoni and his staff were still coping with the aftermath of the Rainbow House fire (Chapter 7). We held our lessons learned workshop in Rwanda in December 2019. My third and final set of site visits were planned to occur in February and March 2020, after the project had concluded. These were interrupted by travel restrictions resulting from the SARS- Cov-2 pandemic. I had visited Côte d'Ivoire and Cameroon in the weeks immedi- ately before my university locked down and international travel restrictions went into place. To the extent possible, I collected what data I could remotely from Jamaica and Zimbabwe. This proved a great challenge. The unstable supply of electricity in Zimbabwe and its routine power shutoffs lasted from the early morning hours until nearly midnight (Banya, 2019). Tools such as Zoom require faster Internet speeds than our partner in Zimbabwe had available. A few quick WhatsApp conversations with Mandla had to suffice. A graduate student and I interviewed Halima from Ghana by Zoom on two occasions to help enrich my understanding of the work there. Akoni, Jaden, Dymond, and I also touched base for the final time by Zoom. In addition, I interviewed MPact staff in January 2019 and May 2020.

My in-person visits typically included observing events, meetings, and activities; touring area health care facilities; holding meetings with representatives of local gov- ernment and community-led organizations; and conducting private one-on-one and small group interviews with community members, project allies and collabora- tors, health care workers, and others who could provide insight on the project ac- tivities and the country's social, cultural, political, legal, and economic context. In the Francophone countries, I was aided by a professional translator (Chantal who attended the Cambodia workshop) or by bilingual community members (Laurent and another community member). All were chosen by our local partner and carefully trained in research and confidentiality protections by me. Chantal also coached Laurent and my other translator on the basics of translation by phone. My visit procedures were adapted in consultation with each partner to minimize the possibility that the evaluation and my presence might undermine the safety and security of those to whom I spoke. I kept no records of names or locations, excepting government offices and health care facilities, unless someone chose to give me their business card. The cellular, Bluetooth, and wireless connections on my phone and laptop remained switched off in the field, along with those on my fitness tracker. I transferred audio recordings to secure cloud storage nightly and then wiped my audio recording device. I kept a diary and took notes to aid my memory, but I waited until I was in flight to elaborate my cryptic scribblings.

When I returned from each visit, I debriefed the country lead verbally and in writing immediately. At times, I spoke with them by phone from in country. I typically did this when something I observed worried me or required clarification. I debriefed the local staff before I departed and shared my written summary with them by email within a few days of my arrival home. After each of the first two sets of visits were complete, I flew to Oakland and led facilitated exercises with the MPact team to make sense of the findings and generate recommendations, including for the evaluation. I used techniques such as hosting a data placemat luncheon.[4] When I used a technique like data placemats, I also created placemats for each of the partners I had visited. I brought those placemats with me on my next site visit. Whenever I could, I introduced simple techniques to MPact and the partners to support evidence-based learning that they might easily integrate into their work in the future. I wrote reports at three points in time, informed by the data and the in-person interactive sessions we held throughout the process.

In addition to the site visits, I surveyed the staff in the partner agencies on their advocacy capacity in spring of 2019, using our original set of advocacy principles as item stems. Ratings were made on a scoring rubric that ranged from novice to expert. The survey data were fed back, along with the first round of site visit data to the MPact team, and to the partners. Importantly, these data affirmed the accuracy of our intuitive placement of organizations into cells for the purposes of sampling. They also provided partners and country leads guidance on partners' most acute needs for technical support and professional development. I observed and interacted with MPact staff in multiple meetings throughout the project, including attending their annual strategic planning retreat in January 2019. With Stephen, Omar, Greg, and Mohan, I co-designed and co-le the 3-day reflection and lessons learned workshop we held in Rwanda for all our partners. I used that occasion to discuss achievements and challenges experienced by our partners from Burundi, Ghana, and República Dominicana. Many of the techniques we implemented in Rwanda I intentionally chose because of their value in generating additional evaluation data and because they could be readily used by the partners in their future work. These included a variation on most-significant-change storytelling (Davies & Dart, 2005),[5] drawing activities, and an appreciative inquiry exercise designed to elicit a list of the conditions that were present when the partners accomplished their best work (Coghlan et al., 2003).

In all, excluding informal interviews with health care providers, journalists, and government representatives during onsite tours and meetings, 112 people participated in a formal semistructured individual or small-group interview; 21 of these people I interviewed twice and 3 of these people I interviewed on three occasions. The people I interviewed more than once are almost exclusively staff members at MPact, a partner agency, or a local in-country collaborator. In Cameroon and Côte d'Ivoire, I was permitted repeated audiences with two high-ranking government officials, one of whom granted me private interviews. Overall, 31.2% of people I interviewed ($n = 35$) were staff members at MPact or one of the seven partner organizations, 31.2% ($n = 35$) were community members, 14.3% ($n = 16$) were staff in collaborating allied organizations, and 14.3% ($n = 16$) were health care professionals. The remaining interviewees were journalists ($n = 4$; 3.5%) or government officials ($n = 6$; 5.3%). (See Table A.1.)

I harvested outcomes throughout the process of collecting data. Consistent with the approach, I defined an outcome as a change observed in a person, group of persons, or an institution that reflected progress toward (or away from) rights-based access to affirming HIV health care for gay and bisexual men and transgender women, and to which Project ACT directly or indirectly contributed (Wilson-Grau, 2018). I looked for changes that could enable gay and bisexual men and transgender women access to health care free of discrimination, stigma, and violence. I also looked for changes that, despite the best of intentions, undercut or impaired the ability of gay and bisexual men and transgender women to exercise their right to access

Table A.1 Project ACT Evaluation Data Sources

Stakeholder Group	Individual and Small-group Interviews	Observations	Archives	Surveys
MPact	•	•	•	
Lead collaborating Partners	•	•	•	•
Medical community	•	•		
Government officials	•	•		
Media	•	•		
LGBTQI organizations	•	•	•	
LGBTQI constituents	•	•		
Other civil society Organizations	•	•		
TOTAL	112 interviewees	68 days	107 documents	33 surveys

nondiscriminatory health care or that undermined their safety. I identified most out-comes during interviews or through observation. Some outcomes proved easier to substantiate through independent sources than others. For example, I verified some outcomes through newspaper articles. I verified some through direct observation. Others I verified through corroboration. Any outcome I could not verify beyond a reasonable doubt, I discarded.

I used principles-focused evaluation (Patton, 2018) to explore the extent to which the advocacy and technical assistance principles the staff and I had articulated at the outset were applied throughout Project ACT and were useful in attaining results. I looked for principles we had not articulated. In Rwanda, one of the exercises we conducted focused on principles. In that exercise, we engaged the partners in iden-tifying which principles they believed were evident in the project and useful, and which were missing. The very last session I held with the MPact team occurred in the late summer of 2020. That session focused on an overall assessment of the project—what we liked, loved, lacked, and learned. The MPact team generated a set of concrete actions they would take to build on the lessons of Project ACT for their future work. This list spanned monitoring and evaluation practices, site visit policies and practices, partnership practices, and project planning practices, among others.

The sum of the evaluation data—interviews, observations, photos, field notes, and archives—and the interpretations that the entire Project ACT team made of them throughout our years of work together provide the basis of the story of Project ACT's implementation George and I tell in these pages. Any errors and omissions in reporting the story of Project ACT that result from the quality of its evaluation are solely my responsibility.

Notes

Introduction

1. Human rights organizations, including Human Rights Watch and the International Federation for Human Rights, are among the online sources providing coverage of this story. Human Rights Watch reported on these events in its annual world report on human rights for 2018 (Human Rights Watch, 2019a). The International Federation of Human Rights posted coverage of these events in an online article dated April 30, 2018.

2. In this book, we use "sexual minority" as an umbrella term to refer to all individuals whose sexual attractions include people of their same sex. We similarly use "gender minority" to refer to those whose gender identity differs from the sex that they were assigned at birth, or whose gender expression does not conform to dominant cultural norms. We use the terms "lesbian," "gay," "bisexual," and "transgender," or the acronym "LGBT" when referring to those sexual and gender minority people who express these identities. We typically use these more specific terms when they best characterize study samples or the focus of a piece of scholarship. We quote people who use the term "men who have sex with men" or "MSM" to refer to men who are same gender–attracted and who do not necessarily identify as gay or bisexual. We recognize each of these terms is dissatisfying.

3. Throughout this book, we use pseudonyms for all informants, including public officials.

4. Throughout this book, we use the term "activist" to refer to the leaders, staff, and constituents who participated in the advocacy work described in this book. We recognize that some of these individuals may label themselves differently, choosing to call themselves "advocates." We prefer the term "activist" simply because of its emphasis on the pursuit of structural and social change, which aligns with Project ACT's mission. Some of the activists in this book also work as advocates, most often on behalf of individual patients who were mistreated in the process of pursuing care, or who were harassed, blackmailed, imprisoned, or violently attacked.

5. We use the terms "inequity" and "inequality" throughout this book, as well as the converse of these terms, "equity" and "equality." When we use "inequality," we use the term to refer to differences between people or groups that are preventable. When we use the term "inequity," we also refer to avoidable differences between groups of people but also to the fact that inequities are unjust or unfair differences. "Equity" refers to providing the resources needed to attain an equal outcome, in recognition of differing circumstances. "Equality" refers to providing the same resources and opportunities regardless of circumstances.

6. These figures reflect data reported by UNAIDS as of April 28, 2023.

7. Community psychologist Ann Brodsky, and her translator and guide to the workings of an underground activist and humanitarian organization of Afghan women (Brodsky & Faryal, 2006), write about the wisdom of not viewing all differences as appropriate or possible to bridge. Honoring and respecting diversity, they argue, does not require bridging difference as much as it requires humility in its presence.

8. I have spoken about both growing up on Fire Island and about my mixed-race background in keynote addresses delivered at the 2017 Culturally Responsive Evaluation Association (CREA) conference and at the 2021 Aotearoa New Zealand Evaluation Association (ANZEA) conference. These addresses were later published in ANZEA's journal, *Evaluation Matters—He Take T? Te Aromatawai.*

9. I have written about my identity as bisexual elsewhere yet found my experiences as a queer woman in a homophobic world less salient than my experiences of racism when we started the work that we describe in this book.

10. In a principles-focused evaluation, the evaluator examines which principles of practice provide meaningful guidance in achieving a desired outcome under specific circumstances. The approach is appropriate to complex and dynamic circumstances in which adhering rigidly to a recipe or prescribed set of procedures is not useful or appropriate.

11. Outcome harvesting is an approach to outcome evaluation rooted in the logic of contribution rather than attribution. The evaluator works backward, much like a detective does in solving a crime, by collecting evidence of what has changed, determining how an intervention may have directly or indirectly contributed to it, and examining its meaningfulness.

12. Our experience of writing this book resonates closely with the experience reported by Alexandra Juhasez and Theodore Kerr in their essay, "Writing is always collective: How we co-wrote a whole book and stayed friends" (Juhasez & Kerr, 2023), https://lambdaliterary. org/2023/03/writing-is-always-collective-how-we-co-wrote-a-whole-book-and-stayed-friends/.

13. In the summer of 2020, the Global Fund made this estimate based on the severity of disruptions to medical supply chains, laboratory functioning, and access to and provision of health care services due to COVID-19.

Chapter 1

1. Portions of this chapter were adapted from an article previously published as Miller, R. L. (2018). Hiding in plain sight: On culturally responsive evaluation and LGBT communities of color. *Evaluation Matters—He Take T? Te Aromatawai, 4,* 5–33.

2. In 2018, history repeated itself. A similar protest erupted over plans to hold the conference in San Francisco in 2020 due to several factors: the unsafe environment in the United States for AIDS-affected communities under the Trump administration; the extreme expense of attending a meeting in San Francisco for participants; and a peculiar plan to situate the main conference in San Francisco itself and to segregate the Global Village a train ride away, under the San Francisco Bay in Oakland, severely limiting opportunities for community engagement in the main elements of the program. Activists voiced concerns about locating the conference in San Francisco at the 2018 meeting in Amsterdam, but to no avail. As part of their boycott, "key population" networks organized and sponsored an alternative conference. MPact was among the leading organizers of this alternative conference.

3. Clinton's address can be viewed at https://2009-2017.state.gov/secretary/20092013clin ton/rm/2012/07/195355.htm.

4. AIDS 2024 reflected a significant departure from past conferences, featuring gay men and transgender women prominently in primary sessions. This conference, however, was also denounced for the failure of the Canadian government to approve visas for prominent

public health experts and activists from throughout the Global South, illustrating the conference's long-standing elitism.

5. The global U = U campaign (which stands for Undetectable = Untransmittable) seeks to educate people that when a person living with HIV takes their antiretroviral medication as prescribed and has achieved an undetectable viral load, it is not possible for them to transmit HIV to others during sex. The campaign began in 2016 as an effort to reduce stigma experienced by people (including sexual and gender minority people) living with HIV, using incontestable evidence about the effectiveness of antiretroviral medications in averting new infections. More information on the U = U campaign may be found at https://www.aidsmap.com/about-hiv/faq/what-does-undetectable-untransmittable-uu-mean and at https://www.hrc.org/resources/u-u-guide-combats-hiv-and-aids-misinformation-stigma-and-discrimination.

6. Although more recent data are available, data for the 2016–2019 period best reflect the state of the epidemic at the time of Project ACT. The most recent data, as of this writing, are that 38.4 million people are living with HIV worldwide and that 40.1 million people have died since the epidemic began (UNAIDS, 2023).

7. In 2016, roughly 70% of people living with HIV were estimated to be aware of their HIV status. About 77% of those people were receiving antiretroviral treatment, amounting to roughly 53% of all people estimated to be living with HIV that year. About 82% of those who knew their HIV status and were in treatment were virally suppressed (roughly 44% of all people living with HIV in 2016). By 2019, an estimated 81% of people who were living with HIV were aware of their HIV status, reflecting substantial gains in HIV testing in just 3 years. Of those people who had learned they were HIV infected, 82% were on antiretroviral therapy, equal to 66% of people living with HIV worldwide. Of those accessing treatment, 88% were virally suppressed, equal to about 58% of all people estimated to be living with HIV at the time (UNAIDS, 2021d). Although there were too many new infections and deaths to meet the 90-90-90 targets in 2018, these indicators of testing, treatment, and viral suppression continued a hopeful downward trend over the decade. However, COVID-19, declining investments, and persistent stigma had undermined this progress by the end of 2021 (UNAIDS, 2022a).

8. Funding directed toward meeting the targets had also flattened (UNAIDS, 2018).

9. By the end of 2021, as we sat down to write this book, "key populations" comprised 70% of the 1.5 million new infections recorded that year (UNAIDS, 2022a).

10. Many people find the term "key populations" offensive and dehumanizing because it can render gender and sexual minority people, sex workers, and people who use drugs invisible.

11. Europe and Central Asia (99%); Middle East and North Africa (97%); Western and Central Europe and North America (96%); Asia and Pacific (98%); Latin America (77%); Western and Central Africa (69%); Caribbean (60%); Eastern and Southern Africa (28%).

12. Unsurprisingly, then, when UNAIDS unveiled its new global strategic plan in early 2021, that plan focused even more forcefully on ending inequity to bring about an end to the HIV epidemic, eliminating the stigma and discrimination that impede public health progress, and advancing human rights as a public health priority (UNAIDS, 2020d). The new plan no longer accepts average attainment of goals across a nation's population, and it sets ambitious targets for country-level enabling environments (UNAIDS, 2021e). The new plan sets explicit benchmarks for the elimination of stigma and discrimination at the

population and country levels, benchmarks that will be difficult to attain given the entrenched state of stigma and discrimination faced by people affected by HIV today.

13. During the writing of this book, Uganda stiffened its criminalization law dramatically (Madowo & Nicholls, 2023), and shut down LGBT-community-led organizations, including the oldest organization in the country, SMUG. Ghana moved toward passing a similarly severe law. Other countries in the Senegambia region also entertained severe laws.

14. The imprisonment and conviction of transgender women Shakiro and Patricia in Cameroon provides an example of the use of misgendering to violate human rights: https:// www.hrw.org/news/2021/04/14/cameroon-wave-arrests-abuse-against-lgbt-people

15. Uganda's recent law imposes the death penalty for those convicted of "aggravated homosexuality," which is defined as engaging in same-sex sexual interactions as a person living with HIV.

16. The African diaspora are the communities of people descended from Africa brought to the Americas via the North Atlantic slave trade. This has been declared the sixth region of the African Union.

17. The most recent UNAIDS data for sub-Saharan Africa indicate that "key populations" comprise 51% of new HIV infections in the region.

18. Cameroon's Anglophone guerilla insurgency was rapidly escalating toward what would become the Ambazonian War, a bloody civil conflict between Anglophone separatists and the state. In the 3 months leading up to our interview, the political crises in the country had taken a severe turn, characterized by intensifying horrific violence and civilian massacres in the northwest region of the country.

19. UNAIDS (2022b) defines community-led responses as "actions and strategies that seek to improve the health and human rights of their constituencies, that are specifically informed and implemented by and for communities themselves and the organizations, groups, and networks that represent them."

Chapter 2

1. Conversion therapy, sometimes also called reparative therapy, refers to efforts to suppress or change sexual orientation, sexual attraction, or gender expression. These nontherapeutic interventions have been shown to cause significant harm and to be ineffective.

2. Evidence from Uganda, following its passage of a similarly vicious law, shows a dramatic increase in violence, evictions, loss of employment, and loss of health care among people suspected of being sexual and gender minorities.

3. The introduction of this bill followed immediately on the heels of high-profile acts of repression in the country and attempts to restrict the participation in civil society of sexual and gender minority people and their allies. In May 2021, 21 human rights activists were imprisoned for 3 weeks without bail on charges of unlawful assembly. The activists had attended a training session at a local hotel focused on how to document and report on sexual and gender minority human rights violations. The activists' eventual release resulted only after strong pressure was applied on the Ho High Court. International human rights protectors, Ghanaian civil society institutions, LGBT community members and their allies, and a team of human rights lawyers raised funds, wrote public statements, and mounted legal arguments for the activists' release, activities that the "Promotion of Proper Human Sexual Rights and Ghanian Family Values Bill" would prohibit. In 2020, the Pan African

Regional Conference sponsored by the International Lesbian, Gay, Bisexual, Trans, and Intersex Association was moved from Ghana after President Akufo-Addo was accused of bringing "a curse" on the country by permitting it. In a radio interview, National Democratic Congress leader Dr. Hanna Louisa Bissiw framed her objections to the conference: "The visionless president wants to bring gays and lesbians to the country to influence our young one into that bad act ... Homosexuality is a disease. In veterinary, you don't have to condone homosexuality; you have to kill all animals that attempt same-sex mating. Why should humans do that?"

4. The chair of Advocates for Christ-Ghana coauthored the bill. Its promoters include the Christian Council of Ghana and the United States–based far-right extremist hate group, World Congress of Families, whose influence in Africa is startlingly powerful (Human Rights Campaign, 2015; Southern Poverty Law Center, 2015).

5. See Chapter 1, note 5.

6. Notable exceptions include indigenous writers.

7. Indigenous philosopher Kyle Whyte describes an Indigenous concept akin to African framings of human rights. Rooted in the language of communal kinship, he suggests communal life depends on fulfilling responsibilities for mutual caretaking (Whyte, 2021).

8. In March 2023, the government of Uganda passed as law a bill containing similar provisions to the bill pending in the Ghanian parliament, provoking alarm among human rights and HIV activists and the global HIV community.

9. It is unsurprising that state actions to harass and intimidate civil society groups addressing sexual and gender minority rights escalated dramatically between March 2020 and the present, sometimes under the guise of enforcement of COVID-19 precautions (Amnesty International, 2021; Human Rights Watch, 2021). Cameroon and Zimbabwe are among the countries in the Global South where reports of increased harassment of sexual and gender minority civil society organizations and activists have risen sharply since COVID-19 lockdowns began.

10. Mitchell and colleagues (2020) also take a critical view of the ability of the transnational nongovernment organization to advance social change in meaningful ways.

11. In the annex on how the evaluation was planned, we describe how we articulated an initial set of principles to guide our collective work, principles which we subjected to empirical scrutiny in our evaluation.

Chapter 3

1. MPact Global Action for Gay Men's Health and Rights was founded as the Global Forum on MSM and HIV also known as MSMGF. It changed its name in 2016 in a deliberate effort to shed the MSM acronym.

2. In December 2023, Burundian President Evariste Ndayishimiye called on the country's citizens to stone LGBT people during a press conference, escalating violence against sexual and gender minority citizens.

Chapter 4

1. Organizations Thomann studied, Alternative Côte d'Ivoire and Arc-en-Ciel, are each by coincidence partners of Project ACT.

2. The post-it notes to which Thomann refers still cover the walls of Alternative's current offices.

3. The term "bird-dogging" refers to getting a duty bearer to state a position on the record by posing a well-crafted question at an opportune moment when they are in public. See Bird-dogging Guide: Get them on the record: https://indivisible.org/resource/bird-dogging-guide-get-them-record and Bird-dogging 101: Use your voice to get answers from policymakers: https://www.amsa.org/wp-content/uploads/2015/03/Birddogging 101.doc.

4. For a discussion of the causal logics used in evaluation, see Gates and Dyson (2017).

5. An intense period debrief follows the procedures of a structured discussion or focus group and is timed to occur immediately after a period of intensive activity to capture information on the context surrounding the intense period, what happened during it, outcomes, and changes in strategies and tactics based on what was learned in that period. A critical incident timeline depicts actions and achievements over time. Media tracking is a method of systematically documenting how issues are being covered in public media.

6. The retreat had originally been scheduled for mid-May in Santo Domingo, República Dominicana, but securing visas for our partners in Africa turned out to be far too difficult and long a process. Visas to Cambodia were quick and easy to obtain, and MPact had strong connections in the country. Moving the meeting 10,176 miles to the east solved the logistical problems for getting the partners all in one place. However, this proved the first of many occasions where the nimble nature of MPact's policies and practices, designed to support advocacy and enable staff to capitalize on spontaneous opportunities, proved woefully misaligned with the slow and bureaucratic nature of Michigan State University and its policies. MSU requires travel authorizations be obtained at least 2 weeks before travel. I had purchased tickets to Santo Domingo just under the wire. Although MSU is unfriendly to anything done at the last minute, Project ACT taught me how to suffer through the occasions where university policy made the work more difficult and led to missed opportunities, such as not being able to contribute to an MPact effort to generate demand for PrEP in Africa, Asia, and the Caribbean.

7. Since departing Cambodia, the staff had impaneled a 14-person international planning committee, recruited a dozen expert coaches, assembled plenary panelists, raised the funds to cover the costs of the day, managed the review of 38 innovative global proposals and the process of whittling them down to a pool of 12 finalists, managed the logistics of bringing these youth to Amsterdam, and arranged a meeting of nearly 300 attendees, in addition to the activities associated with their exhibit booth, events in the Global Village, and their IAS conference sessions.

8. To their point, global surveys of national values highlight the cleavages between the Global North and South on the very issues Project ACT will confront. The Ingelhart-Welzel World Cultural Map (2020), for instance, arrays countries in clusters along two value dimensions. This map, based on a world values survey, places the countries in Project ACT in a cluster emphasizing traditional over secular values, and economic and physical survival considerations over individual self-expression. Openness to LGBT rights agendas is among the defining features of countries that embrace the value of self-expression. English-speaking countries, such as the United States, sit at quite a distance from the Project ACT countries on these two value dimensions. Protestant European countries are farther still.

Chapter 5

1. "Chomma" is a slang term that refers to the perineum.
2. When Promise, Mbuso, Mandla, and I joined the nurses and other staff for lunch in the outdoor courtyard after the training, Mbuso repeated to me the pieces of Promise's story told in Ndbele.
3. Our partners prefer to use the term "self-stigma." We chose to use the term "internalized stigma" only because it reflects the scientific consensus that this form of stigma results from stigmatizing forces that emanate from outside the individual.
4. See also recent research by Jackson and colleagues (2023) documenting homophobic and abusive experiences reported by gay men in Jamaica's institutions of higher education.
5. Patient charters of rights are intended as mechanisms to improve patient care. They do not establish legal rights but provide a framework through which patient concerns and complaints can be resolved and to guide continuous improvements in health care services. Patient charters of rights are paper tigers unless systems are in place to evaluate and seek redress of violation of patient rights and patients choose to access those systems.
6. The data to which Akoni refers are described in McFee and Galbraith (2016) and Smith (2018).
7. The quadrant model distinguishes among sex as a biological concept, gender as a social concept, orientation as a set of attractions and feelings, and sexual practices as a set of pleasurable behaviors.
8. TransWave's relationship to J-FLAG is like the relationship the collectives have to Zimbabwe's Sexual Rights Centre. At the time of Project ACT, J-FLAG provided office space, capacity development, and a financial home to TransWave. J-FLAG bears a similar relationship to another smaller organization focused on the lesbian and bisexual women's agenda called WeChange. Both groups help J-FLAG deepen its relationships to these communities and expand its constituent network.
9. Space rental is a perennial challenge for J-FLAG, especially in areas outside of Kingston. On my second visit, I was to join the staff at an all-day health fair that had been widely publicized. The venue owner pulled out of the contract a day before the event once he discovered its focus on LGBT people. With too little time to identify an alternative location, the event was cancelled at the last minute.
10. In Burundi, the infrastructure to collect this information via cellular phones was developed but had not yet been implemented by the conclusion of the project.
11. The mystery patient approach was used in this classic form in Cameroon, where Affirmative Action established partnerships with nine smaller community-led organizations, each of which drew upon their staffs and members to act as mock patients. Roughly 60% of 30 people who served in the mystery patient role were cisgender gay and bisexual men and the remaining 40% were transgender or gender nonconforming. Mystery patients were trained and supervised by a professional health care watchdog organization. Over a period of roughly 12 months, the Cameroonian mystery patients made 162 covert visits to three high-volume HIV outpatient facilities located in high HIV-prevalence health districts in Cameroon's capital city. Their visits followed a carefully constructed sampling protocol of 54 visits in each of three 2-month-long periods. The 18 people who made visits in each of these time periods visited all three facilities, typically in a single day, seeking HIV testing or a sexually transmitted infection consultation. Two of three facility heads

were aware of mystery patient activity, but employees from security guards to registration clerks to nurses to pharmacists to payment clerks were not. A comprehensive structured reporting tool designed in collaboration with the watchdog organization was completed after each visit. In other countries, community-developed variations of the approach were implemented. In Ghana, our partner's strategy emphasized narrative story collection from 45 mystery patients and from 20 men who had attended one of the empowerment work-shops and who later sought HIV-related health care services. The mystery patients were deployed first to document the quality of the services they received and incidents of stigma or discrimination in a sample of clinics in four health areas. Data were collected in each clinic over a 3-day period. After that, actual patients volunteered narrative reports of their patient experiences using the same narrative guidance. In Zimbabwe, rather than use a classic mystery patient strategy, the Sexual Rights Centre relied on a system of community data collection in which constituents were coached through the process of completing a community-developed stigma checklist after they received care at either of the two health care facilities providing comprehensive HIV services in Bulawayo.

Chapter 6

1. Although community-led organizations in Cameroon author annual reports on acts of vi-olence and other human rights violations reported to them, these data are not necessarily specific to the issues of access to health care. There are large, funded research projects operated by international research teams collecting data on stigma and HIV health care among gay and bisexual men in Cameroon and in other West African countries, but these data are rarely if ever shared with community-led organizations like Affirmative Action or reported in ways that are relevant, accessible, and useful. Indeed, when I bumped into the principal investigator of one such project while I was in Cameroon, he mistook Affirmative Action for Alternatives Cameroun, as did his postdoctoral research assistant. The latter organization was assisting them with sample recruitment. Although they each agreed to send me summaries of the Cameroonian data for the purpose of sharing anything of rele-vance with Affirmative Action, I never had a response to my follow-up communications.
2. Restitution is a normative practice among the associations in Cameroon. If a staff member has the privilege of attending a training, workshop, or other conference, it is an expecta-tion that they share their learning with those who do not have the privilege of attending.
3. Matrons are the chief nurse in a health care facility. They oversee the duty rosters of the nursing staff and are tasked with ensuring quality of patient care. They are responsible for infection control, cleanliness, equipment, and supplies, in addition to supervision of nursing personnel.

Chapter 7

1. Coverage of the fire is reported in the national newspaper *The Gleaner* and by sources such as Mendes-Franco. The results of the investigation into the cause of the fire were not de-finitive. It remains unknown if the fire resulted from aged wiring, was set intentionally, or resulted from another cause.
2. During Project ACT, the organization moved to a slightly larger rented home.

3. Studies relying on respondent-driven sampling succeed in recruiting upwards of 800 gay and bisexual men with ease in Bulawayo (Miller et al., 2022; Parmely et al., 2022). The Sexual Rights Centre staff estimates there are at least 1,200 such men living in the greater Bulawayo community.

4. The Centre's funds for Project ACT were paid in US dollars.

5. A disaster in República Dominicana the very same month as the Rainbow House was destroyed, stalled the project's start there. A large plastics factory explosion obliterated and ruined homes and other buildings in the Villas Agricolas neighborhood (Associated Press, 2018; Dominican Today, 2018), including the very health care facilities the Dominican Project ACT team had long courted to get their work rolling.

6. A data placemat session is one of many participatory processes that evaluators use to share evaluation data, gain insight into how an evaluation's stakeholders interpret what is being learned, formulate recommendations, and inform changes to evaluation procedures going forward. In a data placemat session, the evaluator asks stakeholders to sit together at a table as if they are sharing a meal. In advance of the session, the evaluator creates data displays on placemat-sized pieces of paper. Each participant is presented with one placemat at a time. Participants first examine the placemat in silence. They may make notes on it, circling things that capture their attention and writing out their impressions. The evaluator facilitates a discussion among the participants about the placemat using a standard set of prompts. Once the discussion is complete, participants are given a new placemat and the process repeats. For the MPact evaluation, I created 12 placemats based on the data from the first round of site visits, conducted between December 2018 and March 2019, and results of an online survey of all partners. I created a placemat for each site-visited partner, too, based on their data. I facilitated a placemat dialogue with select staff in these countries at my subsequent visit (July through September 2019).

7. Including my visits for the purpose of the evaluation, all but two countries (Burundi, Ghana) had been visited.

8. A second bone of contention concerned the proportion of funding that had been distributed to the partners at the 11-month point. With contracts signed by the end of summer and early fall of 2018, 5 months or more into the initial project period, spending was proceeding more slowly in some of countries than the project officer desired. From MPact's perspective, they had strung along several of the partners whom they had approached about Project ACT in 2016 for 2 long years while waiting for the funds for Project ACT (Chapter 3). They mounted a rapid project startup at an inopportune time relative to the other commitments they (and partners) took on during the wait. They were scrambling. Their partners were scrambling. The MPact staff expected the LGBT program officer to understand that. It was also the case that he believed the project budget was generous, and that MPact had kept too much of the money for itself, views that were closely tied to skepticism about the value implementing partners add to projects such as this.

9. Penya had devised multiple mechanisms to engage her staff and the larger community in collective reflection, solving problems, and establishing a vision. The staff and collective leaders noticed the shift in how problems were approached under her leadership. "When the leadership changed," Mbuso shared, "I felt the difference." I watched Penya gather the staff and collective leaders to sit with her in the morning sun on the front stoop to hold a reflective discussion on their collective work. They hold these reflections every week. They

debate, deliberate, and strategize together. Peter described this new culture of the Sexual Rights Centre as a united and deliberative team in which hearing different points of view and others' ideas is the source of their power and strength. "If there are challenges that we're facing in program implementation, we always come up with strategies as a team," he told me. "And I believe working as a team is a very good strategy on its own. Because you get to hear other people's views."

10. Michigan State University, like most large Research I institutions in the United States with a well-developed international research portfolio, provides a wealth of resources and supports for safety and security that faculty benefit from as a matter of course. These institutional resources were especially important for Project ACT, since the budget for the evaluation was so small that it could not have supported the development and implementation of a safety and security protocol. These resources included Information Technology support for digital safety and legal and medical assistance.

11. Guy from Cameroon once shared with me that he had it on good authority that in his country, President Paul Biya himself made it a practice to stay informed of groups such as Affirmative Action. Guy expressed little doubt that the government was always watching. Although Burundi and Cameroon are perhaps the more extreme in their hostility among the Project ACT countries, police antipathy toward LGBT-led community organizations in these settings is hardly rare (Introduction, Chapter 1, Chapter 2). The declining climate in Ghana (Chapter 2) and aggressive efforts by religious leaders to silence visible activists led Michael, one of the principal activists overseeing Project ACT in Ghana, to seek asylum at the end of the project. Staff at Alternative Côte d'Ivoire disappeared during the project and were believed to have sought asylum.

12. The strain on mental health described by the mystery patients in Cameroon was voiced in interviews by staff and constituents in every country. A community member in Côte d'Ivoire who conducted outreach to recruit people to tell their stories described their work as "painful." "People are afraid, so the work is not easy," she said. "I hear difficult stories. I free myself by crying at night. I take my time for crying." These strains were tolerated best in the organizations that had established a positive, caring social environment, and especially those that worked to establish formal self-care routines, as did the Sexual Rights Centre, and in those that created sanctuary spaces such as Rainbow House.

Chapter 8

1. "PD" and "pédé" are offensive French slang terms. They are like the English terms "fag" and "faggot" but have more demeaning connotations.

2. I was not able to verify that the journalist had started writing the book or what its content might include. Following the procedures of outcome harvesting, I do not count this as a Project ACT outcome, since I was not able to verify it.

3. Unable to secure a safe environment for ICASA delegates in Uganda, the Society for AIDS in Africa revoked the Ugandans' host country status. The conference was rapidly moved to Durban, South Africa. On November 24, 2021, less than 10 days before foreign delegates would board their flights for South Africa, South Africa reported to the World Health Organization it had detected a new variant of COVID-19, the Omicron variant. On December 5, just days before the opening session, the organizers switched to an entirely virtual meeting.

4. The MPact country lead's advice was informed by a curriculum jointly developed by MPact and physicians from Johns Hopkins University's School of Medicine entitled *Promoting the health and rights of gay men worldwide: A handbook for all health professionals*, which was available on MPact's website under the resources tab at the time of this writing. Later adapted by FHI360, the curriculum addresses topics including men's health needs and how providers can create a friendlier clinical environment for gay and bisexual men and adolescents.

5. The data were from 108 mystery patient observations—36 per health care facility—obtained over a period of 4 months.

6. Providers in Ghana also made similar gestures to assist community members avoid stigmatizing waiting room experiences.

7. In his book, *Love falls on us: A story of American ideas and African LGBT lives*, Robbie Corey-Boulet recounts the harrowing experiences of the "Yaoundé 11" who were imprisoned in one of these facilities after a 2005 police raid on the Victoire Bar.

8. The Universal Periodic Review (UPR) is a process through which all United Nation Member States review each other's human rights records over predetermined time periods.

Chapter 9

1. Throughout this chapter, we draw on the observations the Project ACT partners made during their final transnational gathering, a reflection workshop held over 3 days in December 2019 in Rwanda, and on the observations of the MPact team during their last taking-stock meeting held in August 2020.

2. On March 1, 2023, as we sat down to write this final chapter, Uganda's Speaker of Parliament brought a new anti-homosexuality bill to the floor for a vote. Although the country already has a section of its penal code in which a sentence of life may be imposed on people convicted under the law, the current bill is meant to silence dissent and is championed by, among others, President Museveni and Uganda's Archbishop, each well known for his homophobia. Just days before the bill was put up for a vote, President Museveni is quoted in new reports as staunchly in support of its passage: "We are not going to follow people who are lost. These Europeans are not normal; they don't listen. We have been telling them 'Please, this problem of homosexuality is not something that you should normalize and celebrate.' They don't listen. They don't respect other people's views. And they want to turn the abnormal into the norm and force it on others. We shall not agree." The new bill calls for a 10-year prison sentence for same-sex intercourse or for holding a LGBTQ or gender nonbinary identity. It imposes a prison sentence and fine of more than US$26,000 on anyone who "promotes homosexuality" in any form, including renting offices to organizations. The speaker of Parliament called for a vote by show of hands, challenging her fellow parliamentarians that this would reveal to the Ugandan people who is "for homosexuality" (La Jiwe, March 1, 2023). The bill passed into law, setting into motion unimaginable violence, asylum-seeking, and international condemnation.

3. See Miller et al. (2021).

4. At the end-of-project reflection and learning meeting, we held a morning of panel discussions focused on each strategy in which partners who used a tactic, discussed their experiences of it. In addition to our use of a variation of most-significant-change storytelling, the session highlighted how valuable the tactic proved as part of a suite of advocacy activities.

5. All the principles of practice that we identify in this chapter were discussed and endorsed by the Project ACT partners in one of the workshop exercises conducted in Rwanda. During that exercise, the partners identified principles that we had not considered. They also rejected some principles as of minimal relevance. For example, they believed empowerment was essential. They also believed that being sex-positive, while of general value, was not a guiding principle for the specific advocacy pursued in the project.

6. In Rwanda, the last session of the workshop focused on lessons learned and strategies for the future. Informed by their own experiences and the insights gained from one another, the benefit of community inclusion was first on the partners' list of lessons learned.

7. Throughout the project, we also heard loud, consistent complaints of widespread exclusion of and inattention to lesbian and bisexual women.

8. Jada also attended MPact's PrEP demand workshop. She reported learning a great deal about how to design and facilitate workshops from the opportunity. Like Dymond, she knew nothing about PrEP prior to attending.

9. Stickl Haugen and Chouinard (2019) offer an insightful analysis of power within the context of culturally responsive evaluations, including evaluator power.

10. The total Project ACT evaluation budget was initially US$69,000, which is less than a third of its actual cost once in-kind contributions are accounted for. A budget of this size would have permitted a desk review, supplemented by a modest number of interviews, severely limiting our ability to answer questions of keenest interest. The old joke that one can tell research from evaluation by looking at the proportion of the budget devoted to data collection proved a reality in this case, as the evaluation was budgeted at about 5% of the project budget, 2 to 3 times less than what is typically recommended by evaluators.

11. Robin's ability to donate her time is due in no small part to the fact she is tenured and is not reliant on soft money to support her salary during the academic year. Evaluators in soft-money positions, academic or not, would not have been able to donate their time so freely.

Epilogue

1. As we have noted throughout this book, Cameroon is unfortunately a leader among countries that possess an extremely hostile environment for sexual and gender minority people. In 2014, for example, Cameroon is reported to have held in its prisons more people on charges of engaging in consensual same-sex relationships than any other country (L'obervatoire, 2015). Human rights defenders routinely report thousands of violent attacks on sexual and gender minority people each year.

Appendix

1. Meta-evaluation refers to a systematic process of assessing the quality of evaluations relative to evaluation standards, such as the African evaluation standards promulgated by AfrEA (https://afrea.org/) or those developed by other voluntary associations of evaluation professionals around the world, the Joint Committee Standards for Program Evaluation (https://evaluationstandards.org/program/), or the OECD-DAC evaluation standards https://www.oecd.org/development/evaluation/qualitystandards.pdf).

2. Appreciative inquiry is a strength-based approach to organizational development created by David Cooperrider (https://centerforappreciativeinquiry.net/resources/what-is-appre

ciative-inquiry-ai/)and adapted to the context of evaluation by practitioner scholars, including Tessie Catsambas, Hallie Preskill, and Anne Coghlan. The approach relies on a multistep group process in which teams identify the circumstances under which they do their best work (appreciating) and craft a vision of their future. The exercises that are implemented in the approach can be usefully adapted to support evaluation planning.

3. Critical systems heuristics is a framework developed by Swiss philosopher Werner Ulrich (1994) to prompt reflective practice informed by systems thinking. Ulrich's framework is used to facilitate critical analyses and dialogue about the assumptions people make in framing social problems, their solutions, and their evaluation. Key to the reflective process is an interrogation of boundary judgements: those taken-for-granted decisions about which observations and values are relevant to a problem, its solutions, and evaluation, and which are not.

4. Data placemat sessions (see Pankaj & Emery, 2016) are one of many techniques that evaluators have created to assist stakeholders in understanding and interpreting data. In these sessions, the evaluator creates a series of simple placemat-sized data visualizations, one bit of data per placemat. Participants are presented with one placemat at a time. They are instructed to study the placemat silently and are given markers they can use to write or draw on the placemat as they study it. The group is then led through a series of discussion prompts on the placemat's data, before being presented with the next placemat. For instance, in the placemat session I led with the MPact team after our first round of data collection, one placemat presented basic information about who the informants were that I interviewed, which generated a rich conversation about who to sample in future rounds of data collection. Another presented survey results on each partner organization's advocacy capacity rating. A third presented data on the partner organizations, including staff sizes and budgets.

5. Most-significant-change storytelling (Davies & Dart, 2005) is an evaluation approach in which stories of change are collected and analyzed by stakeholders. The approach is useful for identifying unanticipated outcomes and uncovering the values different stakeholders possess about what constitutes meaningful change. In a typical process, expert managerial panels rate which story is the most significant. Some evaluators have criticized this aspect of the technique for failing to upend prevailing power dynamics and empower communities. In Project ACT, partners chose the most-significant-change story through a structured dot-voting process.

References

African Evaluation Association. (2021). *The African evaluation guidelines, 2021 version.* https://afrea.org/aeg/AEG_ENGLISH.pdf

Aggleton, P., & Parker, R. (2015). Moving beyond biomedicalization in the HIV response: Implications for community involvement and community leadership among men who have sex with men and transgender people. *American Journal of Public Health, 105,* 1552–1558.

Aggleton, P., Parker, R., & Maluwa, M. (2003). *Stigma, discrimination, and HIV/AIDS in Latin America and the Caribbean.* Inter-American Development Bank.

AidsFonds. (2020). Fast-track or off track? How insufficient funding for key populations jeopardises ending AIDS by 2030. https://aidsfonds.org/assets/work/file/Fast-Track%20or%20Off%20Track%20report-final_0.pdf.

Aldrich, R. (2003). *Colonialism and homosexuality.* Routledge.

Alinsky, S. D. (1989). *Rules for radicals: A pragmatic primer for realistic radicals.* Vintage.

Al Jazeera. (2021, August 20). Uganda suspends more than 50 rights groups, citing non-compliance. https://www.aljazeera.com/news/2021/8/20/uganda-suspends-over-50-rights-groups-citing-non-compliance

Altman, D., Aggleton, P., Williams, M., Kong, T., Reddy, V., Harrad, D., Reis, T., & Parker, R. (2012). Men who have sex with men: Stigma and discrimination. *Lancet, 3880,* 439–445.

Amnesty International. (2021, January 13). Zimbabwe: Authorities must drop malicious charges against opposition leaders and journalist. https://www.amnesty.org/en/latest/press-release/2021/01/zimbabwe-authorities-must-drop-malicious-charges-against-opposition-leaders-and-journalist.

Annie E. Casey Foundation. (2007). *A guide to measuring advocacy and policy.* Author.

Arensman, B. (2020). Advocacy outcomes are not self-evident: The quest for outcome identification. *American Journal of Evaluation, 41,* 216–233.

Arensman, B., & Van Wesel, M. (2018). Negotiating effectiveness in transnational advocacy evaluation. *Evaluation, 24,* 51–68.

Arensman, B., van Waegeningh, C., & van Wessel, M. (2018). Twinning "practices of change" with "theory of change": Room for emergence in advocacy evaluation. *American Journal of Evaluation, 39,* 221–236.

Argento, E., Duff, P., Bingham, B., Chapman, J., Nguyen, P., Strathdee, S. A., & Shannon, K. (2016). Social cohesion among sex workers and client condom refusal in a Canadian setting: Implications for structural and community-led interventions. *AIDS and Behavior, 20,* 1275–1283.

Arreola, S., Santos, G. M., Beck, J., Sundararaj, M., Wilson, P. A., Hebert, P., Makofane, P., Do, T. D., & Ayala, G. (2015). Sexual stigma, criminalization, investment, and access to HIV services among men who have sex with men worldwide. *AIDS and Behavior, 19,* 227–234.

Associated Press. (2018, December 5). 3 dead, 44 injured in Dominican Republic blast. https://www.voanews.com/a/dominican-republic-plastics-company-blast/4688382.html

Austin, A., Herrick, H., & Proescholdbell, S. (2016). Adverse childhood experiences related to poor adult health among lesbian, gay, and bisexual individuals. *American Journal of Public Health, 106,* 314–320.

Avert. (2020). Funding for HIV and AIDS. https://www.avert.org/professionals/hiv-around-world/global-response/funding

Awondo, P. (2016). Religious leadership and the re-politicization of gender and sexuality in Cameroon. *Journal of Theology for Southern Africa, 155*(Special Issue), 105–120.

Awondo, P., Geschiere, P., & Reid, G. (2012). Homophobic Africa? Toward a more nuanced view. *African Studies Review, 55*, 145–168.

Ayala, G., Arreola, S., Howell, S., Hoffmann, T. J., & Santos, G. M. (2022). Enablers and barriers to HIV services for gay and bisexual men in the COVID-19 era: Fusing data sets from two global online surveys via file concatenation with adjusted weights. *JMIR Public Health and Surveillance, 8*(6), e33538.

Ayala, G., & Santos, G. M. (2016). Will the global HIV response fail gay, bisexual men, and other men who have sex with men? *Journal of the International AIDS Society, 19*, 21098.

Ayala, G., Santos, G. M., Arreola, S., Makofane, K., Garner, A., & Howell, S. (2018). Blue-ribbon boys: Factors associated with PrEP use, ART use, and undetectable viral load among gay app users across six regions of the world. *Journal of the International AIDS Society, 21*, Suppl 5, e25130.

Ayala, G., Sprague, L., van der Merwe, L. L., Thomas, R. M., Chang, J., Arreola, S., Davis, S., Taslim, A., Mienies, K., Nilo, A., Mworeko, L., Hikuam, F., de Leon Moreno, C. G., & Izazola-Licea, J. A. (2021). Peer- and community-led responses to HIV: A scoping review. *PloS One, 16*(12), e0260555. https://doi.org/10.1371/journal.pone.0260555

Banks, N., Hulme, D., & Edwards, M. (2015). NGOs, states, and donors revisited: Still too close for comfort? *World Development, 66*, 707–718.

Banya, N. (2019, August 1). Power crisis turns night into day for Zimbabwe's firms and families. *Reuters.* https://www.reuters.com/article/us-zimbabwe-economy-power/power-crisis-turns-night-into-day-for-zimbabwes-firms-and-families-idUSKCN1UR4SA

Baptiste, S., Manouan, A., Garcia, P., Etya'ale, H., Swan, T., & Wame, J. (2020). Community-led monitoring: When community data drives implementation strategies. *Current HIV/AIDS Reports, 17*, 415–421.

Barasa, E., Mbau, R., & Gilson, L. (2018). What is resilience and how can it be nurtured? A systematic review of empirical literature on organizational resilience. *International Journal of Health Policy and Management, 7*, 491–503.

Beck, J., Peretz, J. J., & Ayala, G. (2015). Services under siege: The impact of anti-LGBT violence on HIV programs. The Global Forum on MSM & HIV. https://mpactglobal.org/wp-content/uploads/2015/12/MSMGF-ViolenceBrief9_Final-120215.pdf.

Beckerman, G. (2022a, February 13). Radical ideas need quiet spaces. *The New York Times.* https://www.nytimes.com/2022/02/10/opinion/radical-ideas-need-quiet-spaces.html

Beckerman, G. (2022b). *The quiet before: On the unexpected origins of radical ideas.* Crown.

Bekker, L. G., Alleyne, G., Baral, S., Cepeda, J., Daskalakis, D., Dowdy, D., Dybul, M., Eholie, S., Esom, K., Garnett, G., Grimsrud, A., Hakim, J., Havlir, D., Isbell, M. T., Johnson, L., Kamarulzaman, A., Kasai, P., Kazatchkine, M., Kilonzo, N., Klag, M., Klein, M., Lewing, S. R., Luo, C., Makofane, K., Martin, N. K., Mayer, K., Millett, G., Ntusi, M., Pace, L., Pike, C., Piot, P., Pozniak, A., Quinn, T. C., Rockstroh, J., Ratevosian, J., Ryan, O, Sippel, S,. Spire, B., Soucat, A., Starrs, A., Strathdee, S. A., Thomson, N., Vella, S., Schechter, M., Vickerman, P, Weir, B., & Beyrer, C. (2018). Advancing global health and strengthening the HIV response in the era of the Sustainable Development Goals: The International AIDS Society-Lancet Commission. *Lancet, 392*, 312–358.

Bertolt, B. (2019). The invention of homophobia in Africa. *Journal of Advances in Social Science and Humanities, 5*, 651–659.

Biryabarema, E. (2021, August 20). Uganda suspends work of 54 NGOs, increasing pressure on charities. *Reuters.* https://www.reuters.com/world/africa/uganda-suspends-work-54-ngos-increasing-pressure-charities-2021-08-20/

Bober, S. L., Michaud, A. L., & Recklitis, C. J. (2019). Finding sexual health aids after cancer: Are cancer centers supporting survivors' needs? *Journal of Cancer Survivorship*, *13*, 224–230.

Brass, J. N., Longhofer, W., Robinson, R. S., & Schnable, A. (2018). NGOs and international development: A review of thirty-five years of scholarship. *World Development*, *112*, 136–149.

Brewer, R., Daunis, C., Ebaady, S., Wilton, L., Chrestman, S., Mukherjee, S., Moore, M., Corrigan, R., & Schneider, J. (2019). Implementation of a socio-structural demonstration project to improve HIV outcomes among young Black men in the Deep South. *Journal of Racial and Ethnic Health Disparities*, *6*, 775–789.

Brodsky, A. E. (2003). *With all our strength. The Revolutionary Association of the Women of Afghanistan*. Routledge.

Brodsky, A. E., & Faryal, T. (2006). No matter how hard you try, your feet still get wet: Insider and outsider perspectives on bridging diversity. *American Journal of Community Psychology*, *37*, 191–201.

Brokovitch, E. R. (2018, December 31). List of alleged homosexuals endangers 82 in Cameroon. *Africa Human Rights Media Network*. https://rightsafrica.com/2018/12/31/list-of-alleged-homosexuals-endangers-82-in-cameroon/

Buckley, J., Archibald, T., Hargreaves. M., & Trochim, W. M. (2015). Defining and teaching evaluative thinking: Insights from research on critical thinking. *American Journal of Evaluation*, *36*, 375–388.

Burger, R., & Seabe, D. (2014). NGO accountability in Africa. In E. Obadare (Ed.), *The handbook of civil society in Africa* (pp. 77–91). Springer.

Burke, J. (2019, January 16). Civilians beaten and abducted in major Zimbabwe crackdown: Activists tell of abductions and beatings during unrest linked to food and fuel shortages. *The Guardian*. https://www.theguardian.com/world/2019/jan/16/authorities-launch-major-crackdown-amid-protests-zimbabwe

Camp, J., Vitoratou, S., & Rimes, K. A. (2020). LGBQ+ self-acceptance and its relationship with minority stressors and mental health: A systematic literature review. *Archives of Sexual Behavior*, *49*, 2353–2373.

Carman, J. G. (2007). Evaluation practice among community-based organizations: Research into the reality. *American Journal of Evaluation*, *28*, 60–75.

Carman, J. G. (2011). Understanding evaluation in nonprofit organizations. *Public Performance and Management Review*, *39*, 374–390.

Carman, J. G., & Fredericks, K. A. (2010). Evaluation capacity and nonprofit organizations: Is the glass half-empty or half-full? *American Journal of Evaluation*, *31*, 84–104.

Castellanos, E., Lankewicz, A., Ogeta, A., Mulucha, J., Reggee, S., O'Connor, N., & Sherwood, J. (2022). Missing: Meaningful trans inclusion in HIV national strategic plans in Eastern and Southern Africa [Paper presentation]. International AIDS Society 2022 Conference, Montreal Canada. https://aids2022.org/wp-content/uploads/2022/08/AIDS2022_abstract_book.pdf

Chakrapani, V. (2021). Need for transgender-specific data from Africa and elsewhere. *Lancet*, *8*, https://doi.org/10.1016/S2352-3018(20)30344-1.

Chilisa, B., & Malunga, C. (2012). Made in Africa evaluation: Uncovering African roots in evaluation theory and practice. The Bellagio Centre African Thought Leaders Forum on Evaluation and Development. https://img1.wsimg.com/blobby/go/b90876f2-ee33-4056-accb-5bf8f67e9b88/downloads/Bellagio%20Report%20_African%20Thought%20Leaders%20Forum.pdf?ver=1627503436543

Chilisa, B., & Mertens, D. M. (2021). Indigenous made in Africa evaluation frameworks: Addressing epistemic violence and contributing to social transformation. *American Journal of Evaluation*, *42*, 241–253.

Chin-Quee, D. S., Cuthbertson, C., & Janowitz, B. (2006). Over-the-counter pill provision: Evidence from Jamaica. *Studies in Family Planning*, *37*, 99–110.

Christens, B. D. (2021). *Community power and empowerment*. Oxford University Press.

Coffman, J. (n.d.). Monitoring and evaluating advocacy: Companion to the advocacy toolkit. *UNICEF.* https://www.betterevaluation.org/sites/default/files/Advocacy_Toolkit_Compan ion%20%281%29.pdf

Coffman, J., & Reed, E. (2009). Unique methods in advocacy evaluation. *The California Endowment.* https://www.alnap.org/system/files/content/resource/files/main/coffman-reed-unique-methods-%28paper%29.pdf

Coghlan, A. T., Preskill, H., & Catsambas, T. T. (2003). An overview of appreciative inquiry in evaluation. *New Directions for Evaluation, 2003* (100), 5–22.

Collins, J. C., Schneider, C. R., Naughtin, C. L., Wilson, F., Neto, A. C. A., & Moles, R. J. (2017). Mystery shopping and coaching as a form of audit and feedback to improve community pharmacy management of non-prescription medication requests: An intervention study. *BMJ Open, 7,* e019462.

Connell, R. W. (2013). *Gender and power: Society, the person, and sexual politics.* John Wiley and Sons.

Corey-Boulet, R. (2019). *Love falls on us: A story of American ideas and African LGBT lives.* Zed.

Coulter, R. W., Kenst, K. S., Bowen, D. J., & Scout. (2014). Research funded by the National Institutes of Health on the health of lesbian, gay, bisexual, and transgender populations. *American Journal of Public Health,* e105–e112.

Currier, A. (2012). *Out in Africa: LGBT organizing in Namibia and South Africa.* University of Minnesota Press.

Currier, A. (2019). *Politicizing sex in contemporary Africa: Homophobia in Malawi.* Cambridge University Press.

Currier, A., & Cruz, J. M. (2014). Civil society and sexual struggles in Africa. In E. Odabare (Ed.), *The handbook of civil society in Africa* (pp. 337–360). Springer.

Currier, A., & Cruz, J. M. (2020). The politics of preemption: Mobilization against LGBT rights in Liberia. *Social Movement Studies, 19,* 82–96.

Currier, A., & McKay, T. (2017). Pursuing social justice through public health: Gender and sexual diversity activism in Malawi. *Critical African Studies, 9,* 71–90.

Curtin, N., Kende, A., & Kende, J. (2016). Navigating multiple identities: The simultaneous in-fluence of advantaged and disadvantaged identities on politicization and activism. *Journal of Social Issues, 72,* 264–285.

Daniel, A., & Neubert, D. (2019). Civil society and social movements: Conceptual insights and challenges in African contexts. *Critical African Studies, 11,* 176–192.

Daouk-Öyry, L., Alameddine, M., Hassan, N., Laham, L., & Soubra, M. (2018). The catalytic role of Mystery Patient tools in shaping patient experience: A method to facilitate value co-creation using action research. *PLOS One, 13*(10), e0205262.

Davies, R., & Dart, J. (2005). The "most significant change" technique: A guide to its use. www.mande.co.uk/docs/MSCGuide.htm

Dean-Coffey, J., Casey, J., & Caldwell, L. D. (2014). Raising the bar—Integrating cultural com-petence and equity: Equitable evaluation. *The Foundation Review, 6*(2). https://doi.org/10.9707/1944-5660.1203.

Denison, J. A., Burke, V. M., Miti, S., Nonyane, B., Frimpong, C., Merrill, K. G., Abrams, E. A., & Mwansa, J. K. (2020). Correction: Project YES! Youth Engaging for Success: A random-ized controlled trial assessing the impact of a clinic-based peer mentoring program on viral suppression, adherence and internalized stigma among HIV-positive youth (15–24 years) in Ndola, Zambia. *PloS One, 15*(4), e0232488.

Díaz, R. M., Ayala, G., Bein, E., Henne, J., & Marin, B. V. (2001). The impact of homophobia, poverty, and racism on the mental health of gay and bisexual Latino men: Findings from 3 U.S. cities. *American Journal of Public Health, 91*(6), 927–932. https://doi.org/10.2105/ajph.91.6.927

Dominican Today. (2018, December 11). Plastics factory at fault in blast that killed 8: Fire dept. https://dominicantoday.com/dr/local/2018/12/11/plastics-factory-at-fault-in-blast-that-killed-7-fire-dept/

Donaldson, S. I., & Picciotto, R. (2016). *Evaluation for an equitable society*. Information Age.

Dovidio, J. F., ten Vergert, M., Stewart, T. L., Gaertner, S. L., Johnson, J. D., Esses, V. M., Riek, B. M., & Pearson, A. R. (2004). Perspective and prejudice: Antecedents and mediating mechanisms. *Personality and Social Psychology Bulletin, 30*, 1537–1549.

Drucker, P. (2021). Changing families and communities: An LGBT contribution to an alternative development path. In C. L. Mason (Ed.), *Routledge handbook of queer development studies* (pp. 19–30). Routledge.

Duchek, S. (2020). Organizational resilience: A capability-based conception. *Business Research, 13*, 215–246.

Dunbar, W., Labat, A., Raccurt, C., Sohler, N., Pape, J. W., Maulet, N., & Coppieters, Y. (2020). A realist systematic review of stigma reduction interventions for HIV prevention and care continuum outcomes among men who have sex with men. *International Journal of STD and AIDS, 31*(8), 712–723.

Dutt, A., & Grabe, S. (2014). Lifetime activism, marginality, and psychology: Narratives of lifelong feminist activists committed to social change. *Qualitative Psychology, 1*(2), 107.

Earl, S., Carden, F., & Smutlyo, T. (2001). *Outcome mapping*. International Development Research Centre.

Enoch, J., & Piot, P (2017). Human rights in the fourth decade of HIV/AIDS response: An inspiring legacy and urgent imperative. *Health and Human Rights Journal, 19*, 117–122.

Epprecht, M. (2008). *Heterosexual Africa? The history of an idea from the age of exploration to the age of AIDS*. University of Ohio Press.

Epprecht, M. (2009). Sexuality, Africa, history. *The American Historical Review, 114*, 1258–1272.

Epprecht, M. (2010). The making of "African sexuality": Early sources, current debates. *History Compass, 8*, 768–779.

Epprecht, M. (2012). Sexual minorities, human rights, and public health strategies in Africa. *African Affairs, 111*, 223–243.

Esala, J. J., Sweitzer, L., Higson-Smith, C., & Anderson, K. L. (2022). Human rights advocacy evaluation in the Global South: A critical review of the literature. *American Journal of Evaluation*, in press.

Eveslage, B. (2016). Sexual health or rights? USAID-funded HIV/AIDS interventions for key populations in Ghana. In J. Gideon & M. Leite (Eds.), *Gender and health handbook* (pp. 539–560). Edward Elgar.

Farmer, P. (2005). *Pathologies of power: Health, human rights, and the new war on the poor*. University of California Press.

Felt, D., Phillips, G., & Miller, R. L. (2024). Tracing the relationship(s) of CRE and LGBTQ+ evaluation. *New Directions for Evaluation, 2023* (180), 57–64.

Figueroa, J. P., Cooper, C. J, Edwards, J. K., Byfield, L., Eastman, S., Hobbs, M. M., & Weir, S. S. (2015). Understanding the high prevalence of HIV and other sexually transmitted infections among socio-economically vulnerable men who have sex with men in Jamaica. *PLoS One. 10*, e0117686.

Figueroa, J. P., Weir, S.S., Jones-Cooper, C., Byfield, L., Hobbs, M.M., McKnight, I., & Cummings, S. (2013). High HIV prevalence among men who have sex with men in Jamaica is associated with social vulnerability and other sexually transmitted infections. *West Indian Medical Journal, 62*, 286–91.

Fitzgerald-Husek, A., Van Wert, M. M., Ewing, W. F., Grosso, A. L., Holland, C. E., Katterl, R., Rosman, L., Agarwal, A., & Baral, S. D. (2017). Measuring stigma affecting sex workers (SW) and men who have sex with men (MSM): A systematic review. *PLoS ONE, 12*, e0188393.

Flores, A. (2019). *Social acceptance of LGBT people in 174 countries, 1981 to 2017.* The UCLA Williams Institute.

Fox, M. P., Pascoe, S., Huber, A. N., Murphy, J., Phokojoe, M., Gorgens, M., Rosen, S., Wilson, D., Pillay, Y., & Fraser-Hurt, N. (2019). Adherence clubs and decentralized medication delivery to support patient retention and sustained viral suppression in care: Results from a cluster-randomized evaluation of differentiated ART delivery models in South Africa. *PLoS Medicine, 16,* e1002874.

France, D. (2016). *How to survive a plague: The inside story of how citizens and science tamed AIDS.* Knopf.

Fredriksen-Goldsen, K. I., Kim, H. J., Shui, C., & Bryan, A. E. B. (2017). Chronic health conditions and key health indicators among lesbian, gay, and bisexual older U.S. adults, 2014–2014. *American Journal of Public Health, 107,* 1332–1338.

Freire, P. (1970). *Pedagogy of the Oppressed.* Continuum.

French, B. Y., Lewis, J. A., Mosely, D. V., Adames, H. Y., Chavez-Dueñas, N. Y., Chen, G. A., & Neville, H. A. (2020). Toward a psychological framework of radical healing in communities of color. *The Counseling Psychologist, 48,* 14–46.

Friedman, S. F., Williams, S. D., Guarino, H., Mateu-Gelabert, P., Karwacyzk, H., Hamilton, L., Walters, S. M., Ezell, J. M., Khan, M., Iorio, J. D., Yang., L. H., & Earnshaw, V. A. (2021). The stigma system: How sociopolitical domination, scapegoating, and stigma shape public health. *Journal of Community Psychology, 50,* 385–408.

Galtung, J. (1969). Violence, peace, and peace research. *Journal of Peace Research, 6,* 167–191.

Gardner, A. L., & Brindis, C. D. (2017). *Advocacy and policy change evaluation: Theory and practice.* Stanford University Press.

Gates, E., & Dyson, L. (2017). Implications of the changing conversation about causality for evaluators. *American Journal of Evaluation, 38,* 29–46.

Glasius, M. (2010). Uncivil society. In H. K. Anheier & S. Toepler (Eds.), *International encyclopedia of civil society* (pp. 1583–1588). Springer.

Glasius, M., Schalk, J., & de Lange, M. (2020). Illiberal norm diffusion: How do governments learn to restrict nongovernmental organizations? *International Studies Quarterly, 64,* 453–468.

The Gleaner. (2018, December 31). J-FLAG's headquarters destroyed by fire. https://jamaica-gleaner.com/article/news/20181231/j-flags-headquarters-destroyed-fire

Gosine, A. (2021). Rescue and real love: Same-sex desire in international development. In C. L. Mason (Ed.), *Routledge handbook of queer development studies* (pp. 193–208). Routledge.

Gutman, A. (2001). Introduction. In M. Ignatieff (Ed.), *Human rights as politics and idolatry* (pp. vii–xxviii). Princeton University Press.

Gyamerah, A. O., Taylor, K. D., Atuahene, K., Anarfi, J. K., Fletcher, M., Raymond, H. F., McFarland, W, & Dodoo, F. N. A. (2020). Stigma, discrimination, violence, and HIV testing among men who have sex with men in four major cities in Ghana. *AIDS Care, 32,* 1036–1044.

Hagopian, A., Rao, D., Katz, A., Sanford, S., & Barnhart, S. (2017). Anti-homosexual legislation and HIV-related stigma in African nations: What has been the role of PEPFAR? *Global Health Action, 10,* 1306391.

Hatzenbueler, M. L. (2017). Advancing research on structural stigma and sexual orientation disparities in mental health among youth. *Journal of Clinical Child and Adolescent Psychology, 46,* 463–475.

Hatzenbuehler, M. L. (2018). Structural stigma and health. In B. Major, J. E. Dovidio, & B. G. Link (Eds.), *The Oxford handbook of stigma, discrimination, and health* (pp. 105–121). Oxford University Press.

Hatzenbuehler, M. L., Bellatorre, A., Lee, Y., Finch, B., Muennig, P., & Fiscella, K. (2014). Structural stigma and all-cause mortality in sexual minority populations. *Social Science and Medicine, 103,* 33–41.

Hatzenbuehler, M. L., & Link, B. G. (2014). Introduction to the special issue on structural stigma and health. *Social Science and Medicine, 103*, 1–6.

Hatzenbuehler, M. L., & Pachankis, J. E. (2016). Stigma and minority stress as social determinants of health among lesbian, gay, bisexual and transgender youth: Research evidence and clinical implications. *Pediatric Clinics of North America, 63*, 985–997.

Hessou, P. H. S., Glele-Ahanhanzo, Y., Akedpedjoy, R., Ahouada, C., Johnson, R. C., Boko, M., Zomahoun, H. T. V., & Alary, M. (2019). Comparison of the prevalence rates of HIV infection between men who have sex with men (MSM) and men in the general population in Sub-Saharan Africa: A systematic review and meta-analysis. *BMC Public Health, 19*, 1634.

Hood, S., Hopson, R. K., & Kirkhart, K. E. (2015). Culturally responsive evaluation. In K. E. Newcomer, H. P. Hatry, & J. S. Wholey (Eds.), *Handbook of practical program evaluation* (4th ed., pp. 281–317). Wiley.

Hopson, R. K., & Cram, F. (Eds.). (2018). *Tackling wicked problems in complex ecologies: The role of evaluation.* Stanford University Press.

Hughes, A. K., Harold, R. D., & Boyer, J. M. (2011). Awareness of LGBT issues among aging services network providers. *Journal of Gerontological Social Work, 54*, 659–677.

Human Rights Campaign. (2015). *Exposed: The World Congress of Families, an American organization exporting hate.* Author.

Human Rights Watch. (2008). *This alien legacy: The origins of sodomy laws in British colonialism.* Author.

Human Rights Watch. (2009, April 24). Burundi: Repeal law criminalizing homosexual conduct. https://www.hrw.org/news/2009/04/24/burundi-repeal-law-criminalizing-homosexual-conduct.

Human Rights Watch. (2019a). Cameroon: Events of 2018. https://www.hrw.org/world-report/2019/country-chapters/cameroon#

Human Rights Watch. (2019b, May 30). Zimbabwe: Seven detained after rights meeting: Arbitrary arrests, subversion charges part of broader crackdown. https://www.hrw.org/news/2019/05/30/zimbabwe-7-detained-after-rights-meeting

Human Rights Watch. (2019c, January 16). Zimbabwe: Security forces fire on protesters: End excessive force, investigate deaths and injuries. https://www.hrw.org/news/2019/01/16/zimbabwe-security-forces-fire-protesters-0

Human Rights Watch. (2020). Country profiles. https://www.hrw.org/video-photos/interactive/2018/04/16/sexual-orientation-gender-identity-country-profiles

Human Rights Watch. (2021, April 4). Cameroon: Wave of arrests, abuse against LGBT people. https://www.hrw.org/news/2021/04/14/cameroon-wave-arrests-abuse-against-lgbt-people

Ignatieff, M. (2001). *Human rights as politics and idolatry.* Princeton University Press.

The Inglehart-Welzel World Cultural Map—World Values Survey 7. (2020). World Values Survey: Findings and insights. https://www.worldvaluessurvey.org/WVSContents.jsp?CMSID=Findings

The Innovation Network. (2007). *Data collection for advocacy evaluation: The intense period debrief.* Author.

Institute of Medicine Committee on Lesbian, Gay, Bisexual, and Transgender Health Issues and Research Gaps and Opportunities. (2011). *The health of lesbian, gay, bisexual, and transgender people: Building a foundation for better understanding.* National Academies Press.

Inter-American Commission on Human Rights. (2012). *Report on the situation of human rights in Jamaica.* Organization of American States. https://www.refworld.org/reference/countryrep/iachr/2012/en/97769.

International Federation for Human Rights. (2018, April 30). Cameroon: Arrest and arbitrary detention of five members of the association Avenir Jeune de l'Ouest (AJO). https://www.fidh.org/en/issues/human-rights-defenders/cameroon-arrest-and-arbitrary-detention-of-five-members-of-the

International Lesbian, Gay, Bisexual, Trans and Intersex Association. (2021). Maps—Sexual orientation laws. https://ilga.org/maps-sexual-orientation-laws.

Jackson, M., Jackman-Ryan, S., Matthews, G., & Cadilla, V. (2023). Homophobia in higher education: Untold stories from Black gay men in Jamaican universities. *Journal of Diversity in Higher Education*. Advance online publication. https://dx.doi.org/ho.1037/dhe0000470

Jamaica Observer. (2019, July 1). Research, data collection must account for trans gender people. https://www.jamaicaobserver.com/news/research-data-collection-must-account-for-trans-gender-people/

Janamnuaysook, R., Janthawila, K., Wainipitapong, S., Srimanus, P., Tangmunkongvorakul, A., Ross, J., Sohn, A. H., Mellins, C. A., Wainberg, M. L., Philbin, M. M., & Phanuphak, N. (2022, July 29–Aug. 2). Integration of a peer-led depression screening and linkage-to-care intervention among transgender women living with and at risk for HIV at a transgender-led health clinic in Bangkok, Thailand [Paper presentation]. International AIDS Society 2022 Conference, Montreal Canada. https://aids2022.org/wp-content/uploads/2022/08/AIDS2022_abstract_book.pdf

Juhasez, A. & Kerr, T. (2023). *Writing is always collective: How we co-wrote a whole book and stayed friends*. https://lambdaliterary.org/2023/03/writing-is-always-collective-how-we-co-wrote-a-whole-book-and-stayed-friends/.

Kane, J. C., Elagros, M. A., Murray, S. M., Mitchell, E. M. H., Augustinavicius, J. L., Causevic, S., & Baral, S. D. (2019). A scoping review of health-related stigma outcomes for high-burden diseases in low- and middle-income countries. *BMC Medicine*, *17*, https://doi.org/10.1186/s12916-019-1250-8

Kaoma, K. (2016). Unmasking the colonial silence: Sexuality in Africa in the post-colonial context. *Journal of Theology for Southern Africa*, *155*, 46–69.

Kenworthy, N., Thomann, M., & Parker, R. (2018). From a global crisis to the "end of AIDS": New epidemics of signification. *Global Public Health*, *13*, 960–971.

Kenyon, K. H. (2019). Health advocacy on the margins: Human rights as a tool for HIV prevention among LGBTI communities in Botswana. *Journal of Contemporary African Studies*, *37*, 257–273.

Kerrigan, D., Kennedy, C. E., Morgan-Thomas, R., Reza-Paul, S., Mwangi, P., Win, K. T., McFall, A., Fonner, V. A., & Butler, J. (2015). A community empowerment approach to the HIV response among sex workers: Effectiveness, challenges, and considerations for implementation and scale-up. *Lancet*, *385*(9963), 172–185.

Kirkhart, K. E. (2010). Eyes on the prize: Multicultural validity and evaluation theory. *American Journal of Evaluation*, *31*, 400–413.

Klugman, B. (2011). Effective social justice advocacy: A theory-of-change framework for assessing progress. *Reproductive Health Matters*, *19*, 146–162.

Klugman, B. (2022, January 19). Must we call it "evaluation"?—How "M&E" language can be a barrier to institutionalizing learning. *AEA 365*. https://aea365.org/blog/ol-ecb-tig-week-must-we-call-it-evaluation-how-me-language-can-be-a-barrier-to-institutionalising-learning-by-barbara-klugman/

Kosciw, J. G., Palmer, H. A., & Kull, R. M. (2015). Reflecting resiliency: Openness about sexual orientation and/or gender identity and its relationship to well-being and educational outcomes for LGBT students. *American Journal of Community Psychology*, *55*, 167–178.

La Jiwe, J. (2023, March 1). Ugandan parliament is close to approving repressive anti-gay bill. *Rights Africa*. https://rightsafrica.com/2023/03/01/ugandan-parliament-is-close-to-approving-repressive-anti-gay-bill/#more-14289

Lattanner, M. R., & Hatzenbuehler, M. L. (2023). Thwarted belonging needs: A mechanism prospectively linking multiple levels of stigma and interpersonal outcomes among sexual minorities. *Journal of Social Issues*, *79*, 410–445.

Liambila, W., Obare, F., & Keesbury, J. (2010). Can private pharmacy providers offer comprehensive reproductive services to user of emergency contraceptives? Evidence from Nairobi, Kenya. *Patient Education and Counseling, 81*, 368–373.

Link, B. G., & Phalen, J. C. (2001). Conceptualizing stigma. *Annual Review of Sociology, 27*, 363–385.

Link, B. G., Phelan, J. C., & Hatzenbuehler, M. L. (2018). Stigma as a fundamental cause of health inequality. In B. Major, J. E. Dovidio, & B. G. Link (Eds.), *The Oxford handbook of stigma, discrimination, and health* (pp. 53–68). Oxford University Press.

Lipsky, M., & Smith, S. R. (1989–90). Nonprofit organizations, government, and the welfare state. *Political Science Quarterly, 104*, 625–648.

L'observatoire. (2015). Cameroun. Les défenseurs des droits des personnes LGBTI confrontés à l'homophobie et la violence. *Rapport de Mission Internationale D'enquête*. Fédération Internationale pour Les Droits Humain.

Logie, C. H., Abramovish, A., Schott, N., Levermoe, K., & Jones, N. (2018). Navigating stigma, survival, and sex in contexts of social inequity among young transgender women and sexually diverse men in Kingston, Jamaica. *Reproductive Health Matters, 26*, 7–83.

Logie, C. H., Lacombe-Duncan, A., Wang, Y., Jones, N., Levermore, K., & Neil, A. (2016). Prevalence and correlates of HIV infection and HIV testing among transgender women in Jamaica. *AIDS Patient Care and STDS, 30*, 416–424.

Logie, C. H., Perez-Brumer, A., Mothopeng, T., Latif, M., Ranotsi, A., & Baral, S. D. (2020). Conceptualizing LGBT stigma and associated HIV vulnerabilities among LGBT persons in Lesotho. *AIDS and Behavior, 24*, 3462–3472.

Logie, C. H., Wang, Y., Marcus, N., Leermore, K., Jones, N., Ellis, T., & Bryan, N. (2019). Syndemic experiences, protective factors, and HIV vulnerabilities among lesbian, gay, bisexual, and transgender persons in Jamaica. *AIDS and Behavior, 23*, 1530–1540.

Lorway, R. (2015). *Namibia's rainbow project: Gay rights in an African nation.* Indiana University Press.

Lorway, R. (2017). *AIDS activism, science, and community across three continents.* Springer Nature.

Lovell, J. S. (2016). "We are Jamaicans": Living with and challenging the criminalization of homosexuality in Jamaica. *Contemporary Justice Review, 19*, 86–102.

Ma, P. H. X., Chan, Z. C. Y., & Loke, A. Y. (2019). Self-stigma reduction interventions for people living with HIV/AIDS and their families: A systematic review. *AIDS and Behavior, 23*, 707–741.

Madowo, L., & Nicholls, C. (2023, March 22). Uganda parliament passes bill criminalizing identifying as LGBTQ, imposed death penalty for some offences. *CNN World*. https://www.cnn.com/2023/03/21/africa/uganda-lgbtq-law-passes-intl/index.html

Marsh, K., Eaton, J. W., Mahy, M., Sabin, K., Autenrieth, C. S., Wanyeki, I, Daher, J., & Ghys, P. D. (2019). Global, regional, and country-level 90-90-90 estimates for 2018: Assessing progress towards the 2020 target. *AIDS, 33* (Suppl. 3), S213–S226.

Mayo, C. (1982). Training for positive marginality. *Applied social psychology annual, 3*, 57–73.

McCool, A. (2021, July 2). Major aid donors found to have funded "conversion therapy" clinics in Africa. *The Guardian*. https://www.theguardian.com/global-development/2021/jul/02/major-aid-donors-found-to-have-funded-conversion-therapy-clinics-in-africa

McFee, R., & Galbraith, E. (2016). The developmental cost of homophobia: The case of Jamaica. *Washington Blade*. https://www.washingtonblade.com/content/files/2016/01/The-Developmental-Cost-of-Homophobia-The-Case-of-Jamaica_2016-1.pdf

McGinn, E. K., & Irani, L. (2019). Provider-initiated family planning within HIV services in Malawi: Did policy make it into practice? *Global Health: Science and Practice, 7*, 540–550.

McKay, T. (2016). From marginal to marginalized: The inclusion of men who have sex with men in global and national AIDS programmes and policy. *Global Public Health, 11*, 902–922.

Meldrum, A. (2009, October 13). Gay rights are being debated in every corner of the world. *MinnPost.* https://www.minnpost.com/global-post/2009/10/gay-rights-are-being-debated-every-corner-world/

Mendes-Franco, J. (2019, January 5). After a fire destroys Jamaica's LGBT headquarter, 2019 deemed "year of rebuilding." *Global Voices.* https://globalvoices.org/2019/01/05/after-a-fire-destroys-jamaicas-lgbt-headquarters-2019-deemed-year-of-rebuilding/

Mertens, D. M. (2009). *Transformative research and evaluation.* Guilford.

Meyer, I. H. (2003). Prejudice, social stress, and mental health in lesbian, gay, and bisexual populations: Conceptual issues and research evidence. *Psychological Bulletin, 129*, 674–697.

Meyer, I. H., Flores, A. R., Stemple, L., Romero, A. P., Wilson, B. D. M., & Herman, J. L. (2017). Incarceration rates and traits of sexual minorities in the United States: National inmate survey, 2011–2012. *American Journal of Public Health, 107*, 267–273.

Miller, R. L. (2018). Hiding in plain sight: On culturally responsive evaluation and LGBT communities of color. *Evaluation Matters - He Take T? Te Aromatawai, 4*, 5–33.

Miller, R. L. (2021). Global challenges in securing equity and human rights: Re-envisioning the role for evaluation in the contemporary HIV/AIDS epidemic. *Evaluation Matters—He Take T? Te Aromatawai, 7*, 30–56.

Miller, R. L., & Shinn, M. (2005). Learning from communities: Overcoming difficulties in dissemination of prevention and promotion efforts. *American Journal of Community Psychology, 35*, 169–183.

Miller, R. L., & Tohme, J. (2022). LGBTQ+ human rights evaluation in the global south: Lessons from evaluating Project ACT. *New Directions for Evaluation 2023* (175), 139–151.

Miller, S. S., Mantell, J. E., Parmley, L. E., Musuka, G., Chingombe, I., Mapingure, M., Rogers, J. J., Wu, Y., Hakim, A. J., Mugurungi, O, Samba, C. & Harris, T. G. (2022). Stigma, social cohesion, and HIV risk among sexual and gender minorities in two cities in Zimbabwe. *AIDS and Behavior, 26*(9), 2994–3007.

Mitchell, G. E., Schmitz, P. E., & Bruno-van Vijkeijken, T. (2020). *Between power and irrelevance: The future of transnational NGOs.* Oxford University Press.

Moreau, J., & Currier, A. (2021). Queer dilemmas: LGBT activism and international funding. In C. L. Mason (Ed.), *Routledge handbook of queer development studies* (pp. 223–238). Routledge.

Morfit, N. S. (2011). "AIDS is money": How donor preferences reconfigure local realities. *World Development, 39*, 64–76.

Mousa, S. (2020). Building social cohesion between Christians and Muslims through soccer in post-ISIS Irag. *Science, 369*, 866–870.

Mulé, N. J. (2021). Politicized priorities: Critical implications for LGBTIQ movements. In C. L. Mason (Ed.), *Routledge handbook of queer development studies* (pp. 239–250). Routledge.

Müller, A., Daskilewicz, K., McLean, K. Mmolai-Chalmers, A., Morroni, C., Muparamoto, N., Muula, A. S., Odira, V., Zimba, M., & the Southern and Eastern African Research Collective for Health (SEARCH). (2021). Experience of and factors associated with violence against sexual and gender minorities in nine African countries: A cross-sectional study. *BMC Public Health, 21*(1), 1–11.

Mustanski, B., Andrews, R., & Puckett, J. A. (2016). The effects of cumulative victimization on mental health among lesbian, gay, bisexual, and transgender adolescents and young adults. *American Journal of Public Health, 106*, 527–533.

Muwanguzi, P. A., Nabunya, R., Karis, V. M. S., Nabsiere, A., Nangendo, J., & Mujugira, A. (2023). Nurses' reflections on caring for sexual and gender minorities pre-post stigma reduction training in Uganda. *BMC Nursing, 2023*, 22–50.

Nachega, J. B., Adetokunboh, O., Uthman, O. A., Knowlton, A. W., Altice, F. L., Schechter, M., Galárraga, O., Geng, E., Peltzer, K., Chang, L. W., Van Cutsem, G., Jaffar, S. S., Ford, N., Mellins, C. A., Remien, R. H., & Mills, E. J. (2016). Community-based interventions to improve and sustain antiretroviral therapy adherence, retention in HIV care and clinical outcomes in low- and middle-income countries for achieving the UNAIDS 90-90-90 targets. *Current HIV/AIDS Reports, 13*(5), 241–255.

Namwase, S., Jjuuko, A., & Nyarongo, I. (2017). Sexual minorities' rights in Africa: What does it mean to be human and who gets to decide? In S. Namwase & A. Jjuuko (Eds.), *Protecting the human rights of sexual minorities in contemporary Africa*, 2-12. Pretoria University Law Press.

National Academy of Sciences, Engineering, & Medicine. (2020). *Understanding the well-being of LGBTQI+ populations.* The National Academies.

Odinkalu, C.A. (1999, December 5). Why more Africans don't use human rights language. *Human Rights Dialogue 2.1, (Winter).* Carnegie Council for Ethics in International Affairs. https://www.carnegiecouncil.org/publications/archive/dialogue/2_01/articles/602

Onapajo, H., & Isike, C. (2016). The global politics of gay rights: The straining relations between the West and Africa. *Journal of Global Analysis, 6,* 21–45.

Ooms, G., & Hammonds, R. (2018). The human right to health and global health politics. In C. McInnes, K. Lee, & J. Youde (Eds.), *The Oxford handbook of global health politics.* Oxford University Press. DOI: 10.1093/oxfordhb/9780190456818.013.30

Pachankis, J. E., Hatzenbuehler, M. L., Bränström, R., Schmidt, A. J., Berg, R. C., Jonas, K., Pitoňák, M., Baros, S., & Weatherburn, P. (2021). Structural stigma and sexual minority men's depression and suicidality: A multilevel examination of mechanisms and mobility across 48 countries. *Journal of Abnormal Psychology, 1380,* 713–726.

Pachanckis, J. E., & Jackson, S. D. (2022). A developmental model of the sexual minority closet: Structural sensitization, psychological adaptations, and post-closet growth. *Archives of Sexual Behavior, 52*(5), 1869–1895 https://doi.org/10.1007/s10508-022-02381-w

Pachankis, J. E., & Lick, D. J. (2018). Sexual minority stigma and health. In B. Major, J. E. Dovidio, & B. G. Link (Eds.), *The Oxford handbook of stigma, discrimination, and health* (pp. 477–498). Oxford University Press.

Paluck, E. L., & Green, D. P. (2009). Prejudice reduction: What works? A review and assessment of research and practice. *Annual Review of Psychology, 60,* 339–367.

Pankaj, V., & Emery, A. K. (2016). Data placemats: A facilitative technique designed to enhance stakeholder understanding of data. *New Direction for Evaluation, 149,* 81–93.

Paquette, Danielle. (2021, July 28). Lawmakers in Ghana seek to outlaw advocacy for gay rights. *The Washington Post.* https://www.washingtonpost.com/world/2021/07/28/ghana-lgbtq-bill/

Parker, R., & Aggleton, P. (2003). HIV and AIDS-related stigma and discrimination: A conceptual framework and implications for action. *Social Science and Medicine, 57,* 13–24.

Parmley, L. E., Harris, T. G., Hakim, A. J., Musuka, G., Chingombe, I., Mugurungi, O., Gozhora, P., Samba, C. & Rogers, J. H. (2022). Recent HIV infection among men who have sex with men, transgender women, and genderqueer individuals with newly diagnosed HIV infection in Zimbabwe: Results from a respondent-driven sampling survey. *AIDS Research and Human Retroviruses, 38*(11), 834–839.

Patton, M. Q. (2018). *Principles-focused evaluation: The guide.* Guilford.

Patton, M. Q., & Campbell-Patton, C. E. (2022). *Utilization-focused evaluation.* 5th ed. Sage.

Patton, M. Q., McKegg, K., & Wehipeihana, N. (2015). *Developmental evaluation exemplars: Principles in practice.* Guilford.

PEPFAR (The U.S. President's Emergency Plan for AIDS Relief). (2021, May 3). Burundi country operational plan (COP) strategic direction summary. https://www.state.gov/wp-content/uploads/2021/09/Burundi_SDS_Final-Public_Aug-13-2021.pdf

Phillips, G., Felt, D., Perez-Bill, E., Ruprecht, M. M., & Glenn, E. E. (2022). Principles of LGBTQ+ evaluation. *New Directions for Evaluation, 2022*(175), 15–30.

Phillips, G., Felt, D., Perez-Bill, E., Ruprecht, M. M., Glenn, E. E., Lindeman, P., & Miller, R. L. (2023). Transforming the paradigm for LGBTQ+ evaluation: Advancing a praxis of LGBTQ+ inclusion and liberation in evaluation. *American Journal of Evaluation, 44*, 7–28.

Poteat, T., Ackerman, B., Diouf, D., Ceesay, N., Mothopeng, T., & Odette, K-Z. (2017). HIV prevalence and behavioral and psychosocial factors among transgender women and cisgender men who have sex with men in 8 African countries: A cross-sectional analysis. *PLoS Med, 14*, e1002422.

Pousadela, I. M., & Perera, D. R. (2021). The enemy within? Anti-rights groups and restrictions on civil society. *Global Policy, 12* (Suppl. 5), 34–44.

Prilleltensky, I., & Prilleltensky, O. (2021). *How people matter: Why it affects health, happiness, love, work, and society*. Cambridge University Press.

Rao, R. (2014). The locations of homophobia. *London Review of International Law, 12*, 169–199.

Raynor, J., Coffman, J., & Stachowiak, S. (2021). An introduction to policy advocacy evaluation: The concepts, history, and literature of the field. *New Directions for Evaluation, 2021*(171), 11–18.

Reid, Graeme. (2021, August 10). Homophobic Ghanaian "family values" bill is odious and beggars belief. *Human Rights Watch*. https://www.hrw.org/news/2021/08/10/homophobic-ghanaian-family-values-bill-odious-and-beggars-belief

Reuters Staff. (2014, February 18). Gambia's Jammeh calls gays "vermin," says to fight like mosquitoes. https://www.reuters.com/article/us-gambia-homosexuality/gambias-jammeh-calls-gays-vermin-says-to-fight-like-mosquitoes-idUSBREA1H1S820140218

Rights Africa. (August 2, 2021). Thousands petition Ghana parliament to block "worst anti-LGBTQ bill ever." https://rightsafrica.com/2021/08/02/thousands-petition-ghana-parliament-to-block-worst-anti-lgbtq-bill-ever/

Rodriguez-Hart, C., Musci, R., Nowak, R.G., German, D., Orazulike, I., Ononaku, U., Liu, H., Corwell, T. A., Baral, S., & Charurat, M. (2017). Sexual stigma patterns among Nigerian men who have sex with men and their link to HIV and sexually transmitted infection prevalence. *AIDS and Behavior, 22*, 1662–1670.

Rogers, P. J. (2016). Understanding and supporting equity: Implications of methodological and procedural choices in equity-focused evaluations. In S. I. Donaldson & R. Picciotto (Eds.), *Evaluation for an equitable society* (pp. 199–215). Information Age.

Rosenthal, L., & Levy, S. R. (2010). Understanding women's risk for HIV infection using social dominance the four bases of gendered power. *Psychology of Women Quarterly, 34*, 21–35.

Ross, M. W., Kashiha, J., Misedah, L., Mgopa, R. L., Larsson, M., Agardh, A., & Venkitachalam, K. K. (2021). Addressing the healthcare needs of African men who have sex with men: Barriers to healthcare and promoting HIV and STI treatment in Sub-Saharan Africa. *East African Journal of Health and Sciences, 3*(1), 59–77.

Rucht, D. (2004). Movement allies, adversaries, and third parties. In D. A. Snow, S. A. Soule, & H. Kriesi (Eds.), *The Blackwell companion to social movements* (pp. 197–216). Blackwell.

Russell, G. M., & Bohan, J. S. (2016). Institutional allyship for LGBT equality: Underlying processes and potentials for change. *Journal of Social Issues, 72*, 335–354.

Santos, G. M., Makofane, K., Arreola, S., Do, T., & Ayala, G. (2017). Reductions in access to HIV prevention and care services associated with arrest and conviction in a global survey of men who have sex with men. *Sexually Transmitted Diseases, 93*, 62–64.

Santos, G. M., Ackerman, B., Rao, A., Wallach, S., Ayala, G., & Lamontage, E. (2021). Economic, mental health, HIV prevention and HIV treatment impacts of COVID-19 and the COVID-19 response on a global sample of cisgender gay men and other men who have sex with men. *AIDS and Behavior, 25*, 311–321.

Schlangen R. (2014). *Monitoring and evaluation for human rights organizations: Three case studies.* Center for Evaluation Innovation.

Schlangen, R., & Coe, J. (2021). Radical rerouting: New road for advocacy evaluation. *New Directions for Evaluation, 2021*(171), 71–81.

Schulman, S. (2021). *Let the record show: A political history of ACT UP New York, 1987–1993.* Farrar, Straus, and Giroux.

Schwandt, T. A. (2015). *Evaluation foundations revisited: Cultivating a life of the mind for practices.* Stanford University Press.

Schwandt, T. A. (2018). Evaluative thinking as a collaborative social practice: The case of boundary judgement making. *New Directions for Evaluation, 2018*(158), 125–137.

Schwandt, T. A., & Gates, E. F. (2021). *Evaluating and valuing in social research.* Guilford.

Semugoma, P., Nemande, S., & Baral, S. (2012). The irony of homophobia in Africa. *The Lancet, 380*, 312–313.

SenGupta, S., Hopson, R., & Thompson-Robinson, M. (Eds.) (2004). In search of cultural competence in evaluation: Toward principles and practices. *New Directions for Evaluation, 2004*(102).

Simonovits, G., Kezdi, G., & Kardos, P. (2018). Seeing the world through the other's eye: An online intervention reducing ethnic prejudice. *American Political Science Review, 112*, 186–193.

Smith, A. D., Kimani, J., Kabuti, R., Weatherburn, P., Fearon, E., & Bourne, A. (2021). HIV burden and correlates of infection among transfeminine people and cisgender men who have sex with men in Nairobi, Kenya: An observational study. *The Lancet HIV, 8*(5), e274–e283.

Smith, D. E. (2018). Homophobic and transphobic violence against youth: The Jamaican context. *International Journal of Adolescence and Youth, 23*, 250–258.

Smith, S. L. (2019). Factoring civil society actors into health policy processes in low- and middle-income countries: A review of research articles, 2007–16. *Health Policy and Planning, 34*, 67–77.

Southern Poverty Law Center. (2021). *World Congress of Families.* Author.

Stangl, A. L., Singh, D., Windle, M., Sievwright, K., Footer, K., Iovita, A., Mukasa, S., & Baral, S. (2019). A systematic review of selected human rights programs to improve HIV-related outcomes from 2003 to 2015: What do we know? *BMC Infectious Diseases, 19*, 209.

Stannah, J., Dale, E., Elmes, J., Staunton, R., Beyrer, C., Mitchell, K. M., & Boily, M. C. (2019). HIV testing and engagement with the HIV treatment cascade among men who have sex with men in Africa: A systematic review and meta-analysis. *The Lancet HIV, 6*(11), e769–e787.

Starhawk. (1987). *Truth or dare: Encounters with power, authority, and mystery.* Harper Collins.

Staub, E., & Volhardt, J. (2008). Altruism born of suffering: the roots of caring and helping after victimization and other trauma. *American Journal of Orthopsychiatry, 78*, 267–280.

Stickl Haugen, J., & Chouinard, J. A. (2019). Transparent, translucent, opaque: Exploring the dimensions of power in culturally responsive evaluation contexts. *American Journal of Evaluation, 40*(3), 376–394.

Strömdahl, S., Hoijer, J., & Eriksen, J. (2019). Uptake of peer-led venue-based HIV testing sites in Sweden aimed at men who have sex with men (MSM) and trans persons: A cross-sectional survey. *Sexually Transmitted Infections, 95*, 575–579.

Sundararaj, M., Thapa, S. J., Zah, R., & Mason, K. (2021). *Promoting the health and rights of gay men worldwide: A handbook for all health professionals.* Oakland, CA: MPact Global Action for Gay Men's Health and Rights and Johns Hopkins University.

Suthar, A. B., Ford, N., Bachanas, P. J., Wong, V. J., Rajan, J. S., Saltzman, A. K., Ajose, O., Fakoya, A. O., Granich, R. M., Negussie, E. K., & Baggaley, R. C. (2013). Towards universal voluntary HIV testing and counselling: A systematic review and meta-analysis of community-based approaches. *PLoS Medicine, 10*(8), e1001496.

Teles, S., & Schmitt, M. (2011). The elusive craft of evaluating advocacy. *Stanford Social Innovation Review, 9*, 39–43.

Thomann, M. (2016). HIV vulnerability and the erasure of sexual and gender diversity in Abidjan, Côte d'Ivoire. *Global Public Health, 11*, 994–1009.

Todd, A. R., & Galinsky, A. D. (2014). Perspective-taking as strategy for improving intergroup relations: Evidence, mechanisms, and qualifications. *Social and Personality Psychology Compass, 8*(7), 374–387.

Trapence, G., Collins, C., Avrett, S., Carr, R., Sanchez, H., Ayala, G., Diouf, D., Beyrer, C., & Baral, S. D. (2012). From personal survival to public health: Community leadership by men who have sex with men in the response to HIV. *Lancet, 380*(9839), 400–410. https://doi.org/10.1016/S0140-6736(12)60834-4

Ulrich, W. (1994). *Critical heuristics of social planning: A new approach to practical philosophy*. Wiley.

UNAIDS. (2018). UNAIDS Data 2018. https://www.unaids.org/en/resources/documents/2018/unaids-data-2018

UNAIDS. (2019). UNAIDS Data 2019. https://www.unaids.org/sites/default/files/media_asset/2019-UNAIDS-data_en.pdf

UNAIDS. (2020a). Global AIDS Update 2020. https://www.unaids.org/en/resources/documents/2020/global-aids-report.

UNAIDS. (2020b). New HIV infections increasing among key populations. https://www.unaids.org/en/resources/presscentre/featurestories/2020/september/20200928_new-hiv-infections-increasingly-among-key-populations

UNAIDS. (2020c). New HIV infections among gay men and other men who have sex with men increasing. https://www.unaids.org/en/resources/presscentre/featurestories/2020/december/20201207_new-hiv-infections-increasing

UNAIDS. (2020d). *Seizing the moment. Tackling entrenched inequalities to end epidemics*. Author.

UNAIDS. (2021a). Laws and policies analytics. http://lawsandpolicies.unaids.org.

UNAIDS. (2021b, January 10). Update: Attaining UNAIDS' proposed societal and legal barrier targets could stop 440 000 AIDS-related deaths. https://www.unaids.org/en/resources/presscentre/featurestories/2021/january/20210111_societal-legal-barrier-targets-could-stop-aids-related-deaths

UNAIDS. (2021c). Country factsheets, Ghana 2020. https://www.unaids.org/en/regionscountries/countries/ghana

UNAIDS. (2021d). Global HIV AIDS statistics, fact sheet 2020. https://www.unaids.org/en/resources/fact-sheet

UNAIDS. (2021e). *Global commitments, local actions: After 40 years of AIDS, charting a course to end the pandemic*. Author.

UNAIDS. (2021f). *Global AIDS update confronting inequalities: Lessons for pandemic response from 40 years of AIDS*. Author.

UNAIDS. (2022a). In danger: UNAIDS global update 2022. https://www.unaids.org/en/resources/documents/2022/in-danger-global-aids-update

UNAIDS. (2022b). *Community-led AIDS responses: Final report based on the recommendations of the multistakeholder task team*. Author.

United Nations Population Fund, Global Forum on MSM & HIV, United Nations Development Programme, World Health Organization, United States Agency for International Development, World Bank. (2015, September 8). *Implementing comprehensive HIV and STI programmes with men who have sex with men: Practical guidance for collaborative interventions*. https://www.unfpa.org/publications/implementing-comprehensive-hiv-and-sti-programmes-men-who-have-sex-men.

United States Bureau of the Census, Current Population Reports, Series P-60, No. 162, Money Income of Households, Families, and Persons in the United States: 1987. U.S. Government Printing Office, Washington, D.C., 1989.

United States Department of State. (2016, July 16). Elton John AIDS Foundation and PEPFAR announce inaugural LGBT fund recipients. *APO Group Africa Newsroom*. https://www.africa-newsroom.com/press/elton-john-aids-foundation-and-pepfar-announce-inaugural-lgbt-fund-recipients?lang=en.

Valdesseri, R. O., Holtgrave, D. R., Poteat, T. C., & Beyrer, C. (2019). Unraveling health disparities among sexual and gender minorities: A commentary on the persistent impact of stigma. *Journal of Homosexuality, 66*, 571–589.

Vo, A. T., & Archibald, T. (Eds.) (2018). Evaluative thinking. *New Directions for Evaluation, 2018*(158).

Vollhardt, J. R. (2009). Altruism born of suffering and prosocial behavior following adverse life events: A review and conceptualization. *Social Justice Research, 22*, 53–97.

Vollhardt, J. R., & Staub, E. (2011). Inclusive altruism born of suffering: The relationship between adversity and prosocial attitudes and behavior toward disadvantaged outgroups. *American Journal of Orthopsychiatry, 81*(3), 307.

Wamai, R. G. (2014). Civil society's response to the HIV/AIDS crisis in Africa. In E. Obadare (Ed.), *The handbook of civil society in Africa* (pp. 361–398). Springer.

Watkins, S. C., & Swidler, A. (2012) Working misunderstandings: Donors, brokers, and villagers in Africa's AIDS industry. *Population and Development Review, 38*, S197–S218.

Weerawardhana, C. (2021). Decolonising development work: A transfeminist perspective. In C. L. Mason (Ed.), *Routledge handbook of queer development studies* (pp. 119–130). Routledge.

White, R. C., & Carr, R. (2005). Homosexuality and HIV/AIDS stigma in Jamaica. *Culture, Health, and Sexuality, 7*(4), 347–359.

Whyte, K. P. (2021). Time as kinship. In J. Cohen & S. Foote (Eds)., *The Cambridge companion to environmental humanities* (pp. 39–69.) Cambridge University Press.

Wilson-Grau, R. (2018). *Outcome harvesting: Principles, steps, and evaluation applications.* Information Age.

Wilson-Grau, R., & Britt, H. (2012). *Outcome harvesting*. Ford Foundation.

World Health Organization. (2018). *Focus on key populations in National HIV strategic plans in the African region.* Author.

Yang, F., Janamnuaysook, R., Boyd, M., Phanuphak, N., & Tucker, J. D. (2020). Key populations and power: People-centered social innovation in Asian HIV service. *Lancet, 7*(1), e69–e74.

The Yogyakarta Principles Expert Consensus Panel. (2006). The Yogyakarta Principles: Principles on the application of international human rights law in relation to sexual orientation and gender identity. www.yogyakaraprinciples.org.

Index

For the benefit of digital users, indexed terms that span two pages (e.g., 52–53) may, on occasion, appear on only one of those pages.

Tables and figures are indicated by *t* and *f* following the page number